Hi Gorgeous!

Transforming Inner Power Into Radiant Beauty

CANDIS CAYNE

with Katina Z. Jones

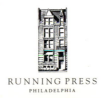

Running Press
PHILADELPHIA

Books published by Running Press are
available at special discounts for bulk
purchases in the United States by corporations,
institutions, and other organizations.
For more information, please contact the
Special Markets Department at Perseus Books,
2300 Chestnut Street, Suite 200, Philadelphia,
PA 19103, or call (800) 810-4145, ext. 5000, or
e-mail special.markets@perseusbooks.com.

ISBN 978-0-7624-6258-2
Library of Congress Control Number:
2017930889

E-book ISBN 978-0-7624-6259-9

9 8 7 6 5 4 3 2 1
Digit on the right indicates the number
of this printing

Designed by Frances J. Soo Ping Chow
Edited by Cindy De La Hoz
Hair: Danna Davis
Makeup: Christian Sanchez
Typography: Adobe Caslon, Archer, Faith
and Glory, and Helvetica Neue

Running Press Book Publishers
2300 Chestnut Street
Philadelphia, PA 19103-4371

Visit us on the web!
www.runningpress.com

Photo credits:
Photography © 2017 Kourosh Sotoodeh except where noted.
p.10 James White; pp 18–21, 23–24, 27–28, 38, 40, 50, 136, 161, 176–177 Candis Cayne;
32–33, 188 experts and designers

This book is dedicated to my mother, Patricia; my father, Gary; and my brother, Dylan, who encouraged me to thrive as my authentic self for my entire life. To my friends and family, who have been my joy and happiness. T, C, C, A, J, M, L, D, J, M, R, A, and J, I love you all! And, finally, to everyone who lives and inspires all in beauty.

—CANDIS

To Harriet, the real beauty expert on my family tree.

—KATINA

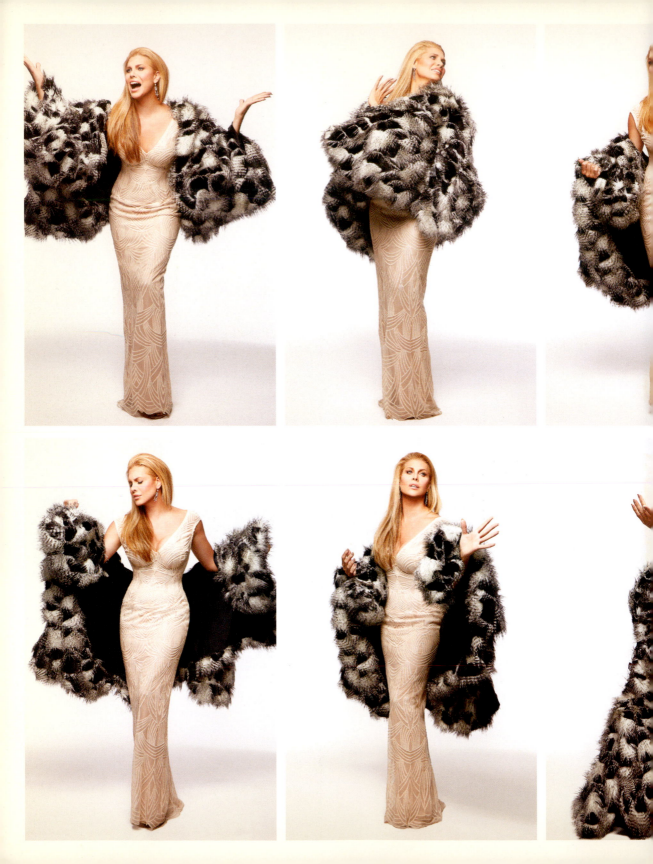

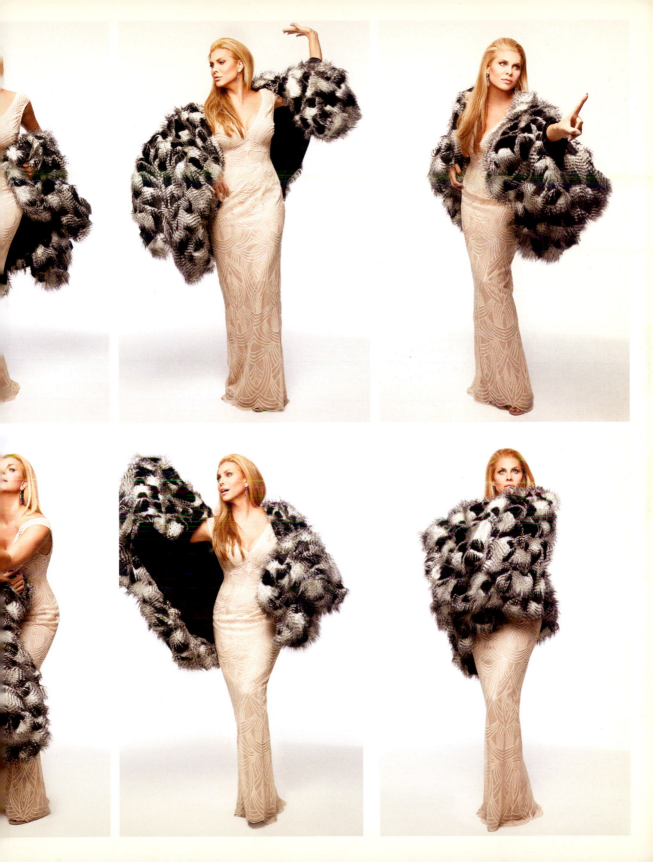

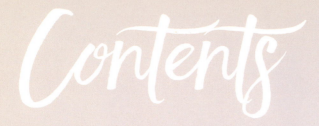

Contents

PART TWO:
GIVING THEM
THE HIGHLIGHTS . 71

CHAPTER EIGHT: NAILIN' IT . 117

CHAPTER NINE: YOUR CROWNING GLORY . 129

PART THREE:
ACCENTUATING
YOUR TRUE SELF. 141

CHAPTER TEN: WHO (AND WHAT)
ARE YOU WEARING? . 143

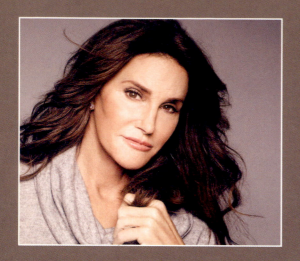

CAITLYN JENNER

Beauty is a funny thing. In Hollywood, we use the word a lot: this beautiful actress, her beautiful dress, his beautiful eyes. But I think everyone somehow knows when they find *true* beauty—the kind that makes you stop in your tracks, the kind that you can't forget. Maybe because it's something you *feel* more than you *see*.

Let me tell you, when you meet my friend Candis—Candis is *beautiful*. It's not her gorgeous hair (though she has that . . . my god, that hair!) or her big almond eyes (she will definitely melt you with those baby blues), but the way her positive spirit infects those around her. It's the way her radiant smile and bubbling laughter make you want to luxuriate in life the way she does.

For many years, before I came out—when I was "stealth Caitlyn"—I tried to follow anyone I could who was trans. Candis was one of them. I mainly knew her because of her show, *Dirty Sexy Money.* I thought, "How cool is that: a trans woman playing a trans character!" She not only looked fantastic, but she looked comfortable in her own skin, comfortable with who she was. Her glow stuck in my mind, so when we were getting ready to select the cast for *I Am Cait*, Candis was first on my list. I didn't get to meet her until right before we started shooting. She waltzed into my house for dinner, flipped her hair, and her smile lit up the room. I wasn't disappointed—she was and is a wonderful, kind human being. I love her style and her beauty, inside and out.

As we've gotten to know each other, I've learned where some of Candis's confidence comes from. It comes from a beautiful soul and many years of purging those voices of self-doubt that say, "You're not good enough, you're not pretty enough, you're not feminine enough." It's a difficult and exhausting task, but when you keep at it, those around you can tell. I believe that beauty comes from within, and that being true to who you are is the best way to project your personal image of beauty.

Another thing I've learned about beauty is that it often shows up in unexpected places. On one of our first trips together, the whole crew headed up to Shelina Moreda's Girlz Motocamp in Napa Valley to learn how to race dirt bikes. When Candis, all geared up in a padded jumpsuit, took her helmet off and flipped her gorgeous mane of hair back, we all cheered. It was completely spontaneous, we couldn't help it! Candis is glamorous against all odds.

Every person deserves to feel comfortable in their body and to face the world with confidence. Who better to serve as an example and to write a book on beauty than my beautiful friend, Candis Cayne, who has mastered this art both inside and out? I truly hope she's able to help you as much as she's helped me because YOU are beautiful, too, and you deserve all the best in life.

Love to you all! And lots of love to my wonderful Candis.

—Cait

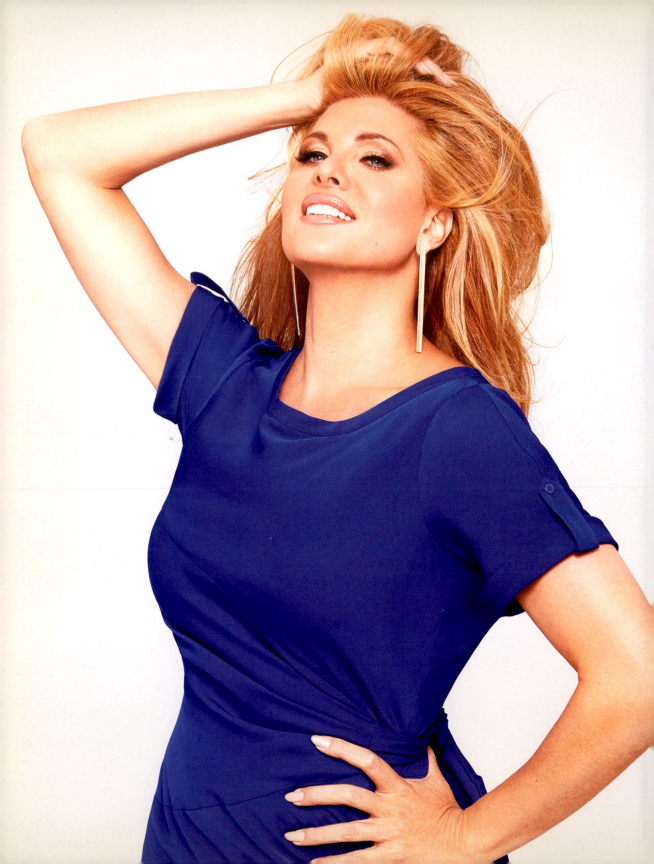

Part One:

Finding Your Inner Radiance

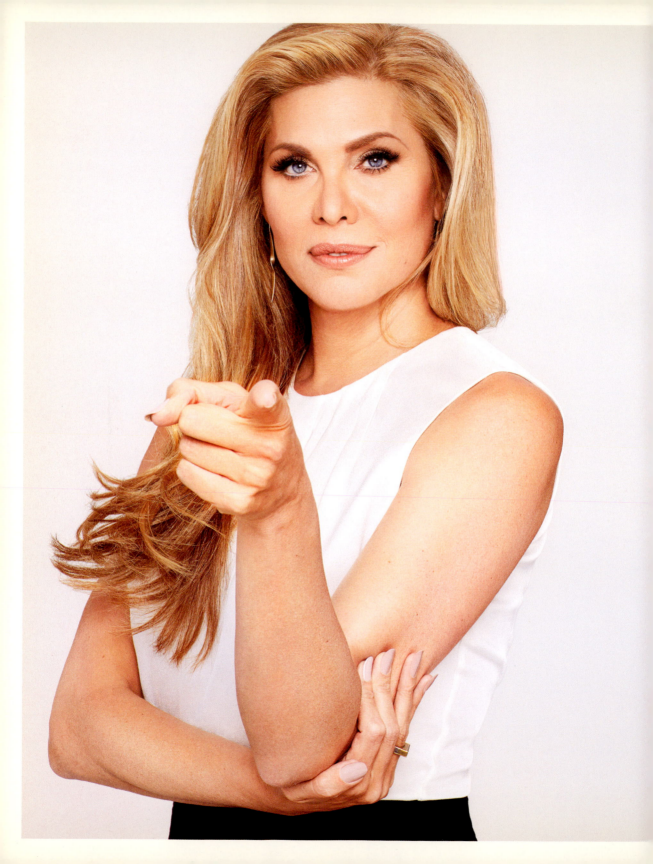

CHAPTER ONE

CELEBRATING YOU

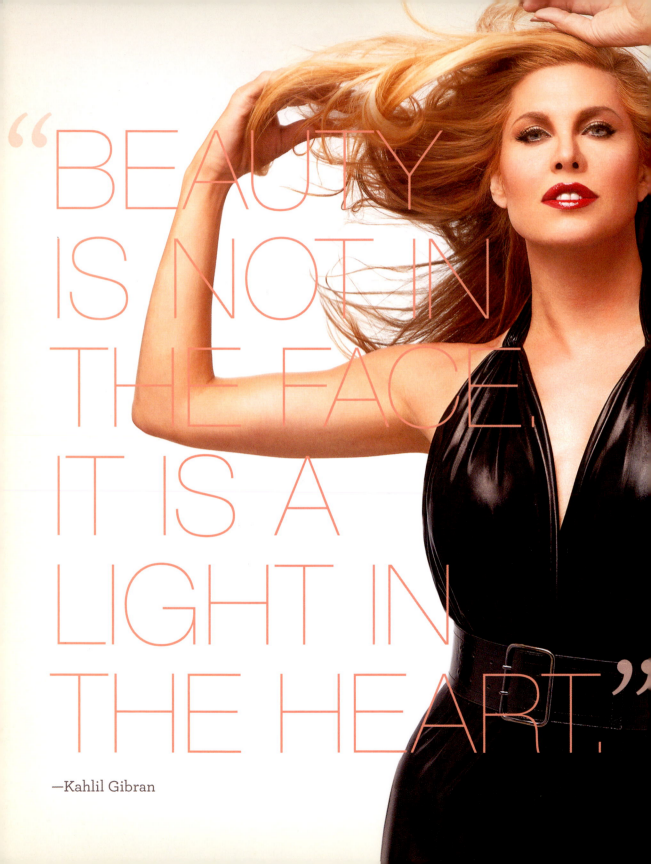

"BEAUTY IS NOT IN THE FACE. IT IS A LIGHT IN THE HEART."

—Kahlil Gibran

So, you've picked up this book, and you're already wondering how this is going to be any different from all the other beauty books out there. Well, for one thing, how many of those books are written by women whose journey to womanhood began after being born into a male body?

Before you slam this book shut, convinced that it isn't actually for you, you should know one more thing: No matter how you define yourself, no matter what type of female you are in your innermost dreams, you *will* see yourself within these pages. This is a book where *all* are welcome, free from fear and shame and judgment. It's about learning not to let those feelings define or inhibit you. This is about expressing your inner beauty!

I'm an actress in L.A., so I am used to living in a skin-deep world where every person is judged on the basis of looks alone. And every day, I see women across the entire spectrum of femininity who berate themselves or allow themselves to think they are "worth less" because they are not built like supermodels. Some of these women are already famous—A-listers who are just as insecure as you might feel at times. Some, like Lupita Nyong'o, have won Oscars before they finally felt like they could own their beauty.

This self-perpetuated, societally reinforced "body shaming" makes me so sad, because the most important thing I've learned on my long journey to womanhood is that you're only as beautiful as you believe yourself to be—and if you don't believe you're beautiful or even worthy of beauty in the first place, you're never going to experience the absolute joy that comes from living a life of radiance, happiness, and especially freedom. How about using that negative energy to your advantage by turning it into your own special power to simply *be* beautiful?

Here's a little secret: We all have the same goals, worries, and insecurities about our looks; however, more important, we share a birthright to be beautiful. What we need is a totally new definition of what beauty actually is so the playing field becomes fuller—more real, well-rounded, and inclusive than ever before—and that's

MY BEAUTIFUL BEGINNING

I grew up in a Hawaiian paradise, surrounded by natural beauty from my earliest days. Still, even when I was a little kid, people would come up to me and ask, "Are you a boy or a girl?" because my feminin-

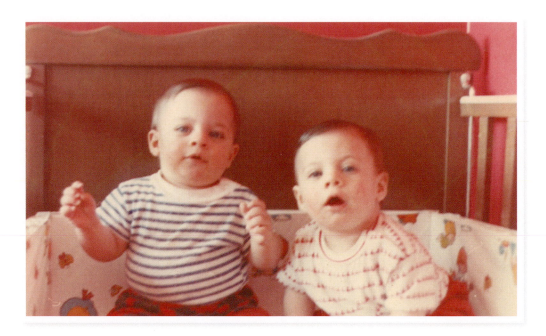

why I've written this book. *For you, gorgeous!* Because each one of us is capable of being, expressing, and living in beauty. Finding and conveying your real self—with confidence—is the key to it all. It's the foundation for every bit of beauty you are seeking to exude. As a bit of a trailblazer myself, I know what I am talking about. Trust me, I've been there!

ity was always somehow visible. It radiates, and comes from the deepest source of my inner being. It's not something that was learned—it was always the most natural feeling in the world to me. I knew in my heart and soul that I was born to be a woman. These feelings, though, confused and angered people, so growing up was not always easy.

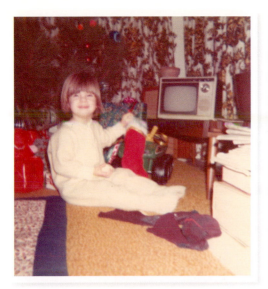

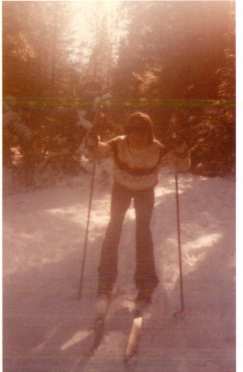

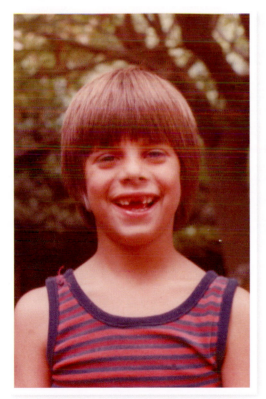

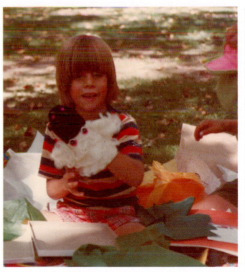

Me and my twin brother Dylan.

Scenes from my happy childhood.

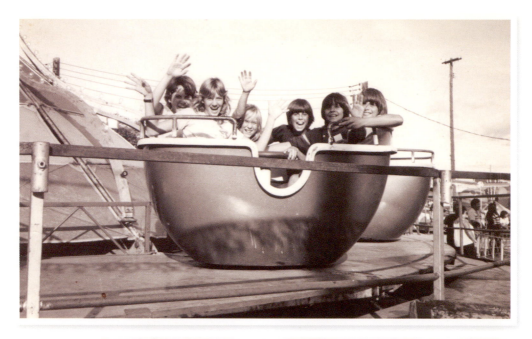

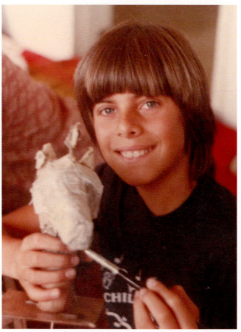

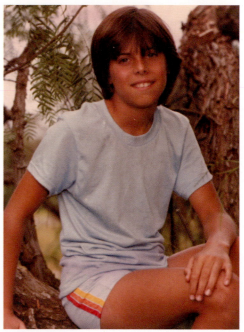

THIS PAGE, TOP: Me (third from left), with my friends Marna, Shawna, Viva, Christian, and brother Dylan.

THIS PAGE, BOTTOM: Me, about age twelve

OPPOSITE: Celebrating my high school graduation with dad, mom, and friends Christina and Eleanor.

My first experience with this was when I moved to Maui and took a family trip to Hana. I saw kids jumping off the Hana Pier into the beautiful blue water and wanted to join in. I ran up and said "hi," then jumped into the water. I looked up with a smile and the other kids said, *mahu* (meaning "faggot"), and started to jump onto my head from the pier. Of course, I panicked and quickly swam to shore, not understanding the name they were calling me nor

very similar. Honestly, it's how you rise above it all and stay true to yourself, no matter how long it takes, that ultimately defines you.

Still, despite all of these feelings, there was no way at that time to research anything, no Internet to rely on for connection with others who felt the same way. It took a much longer time for me to find my tribe than it does for others who identify as female today.

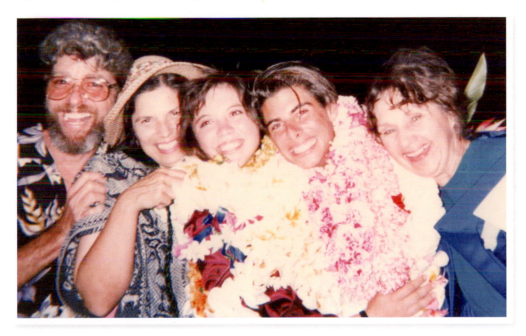

the anger they felt; still, it was the first time I truly realized I was different. This story is not the only one like it over my lifetime thus far, but you know what? We all have a story like this; many of you reading this can no doubt remember something

I knew that I had to leave Maui in order to follow my dream and discover who I truly was meant to be. So, after I graduated from high school, I moved to Los Angeles with $400 in my pocket (much to the chagrin of my parents, because they were so scared for me) and trained as a dancer. I stayed there for one year, got a job dancing on a cruise ship for eight months to save money, then headed to New York City and rented a living room couch in hopes of fulfilling my dreams. I got a scholarship to the Steps dance studio, and worked as a "Kitty Girl" at the Roxy, a former gay club in Chelsea. The gay clubs were where I fell in love with drag. I started to participate in drag shows, but even that was not enough to fully express my true self.

Nothing made sense. I just felt better when I actually *was* female. And I started to think about whose responsibility it really was to express that true inner self—confidently and beautifully. And that thinking changed everything.

START FROM INSIDE

Let's talk more about what it feels like to not feel right in your body, to not be your authentic self. For so many of us, this is a constant thing that plays in our minds, because we tend to spend so much more time focusing on the outside rather than the inside. A lot of us tend to think negatively: If you're single, are you going to attract someone? If married, how will you keep the spark alive? If thin, how can you gain? If overweight, which diet can you try this time?

The trans narrative about this is that we tend to get in our heads questions like, "Am I feminine enough?" and "Am I passable enough?" That can quickly become a mean inner bully. It's an interesting thing to talk about, and it can be something all of us feel for different reasons. For example, if you're African American, there's an automatic "card" you're dealt because of the color of your skin. Or if you're fair-haired, your inner bully may focus on everything being a "blonde thing."

Getting control of your inner critic is all about being able to shut off that inner bully—and start feeding your inner beauty. I work at it, too. I'm not immune, but I've also learned how to use my inner bully inspiration for kinder words: "Okay, so you don't feel great right now. Start working out, start meditating, go to a class and learn something, or just talk to a friend." A lot of times, we internalize all of this pain and don't talk about it to others, and that's what's dangerous, because then you've confined yourself in a hopeless place. But I live by the Golden Rule: "Do unto others, as you would have them do unto you."

I wake up every day and still need to remind myself of the importance of remaining positive in the face of bullies, both inner and outer ones. I think about my best

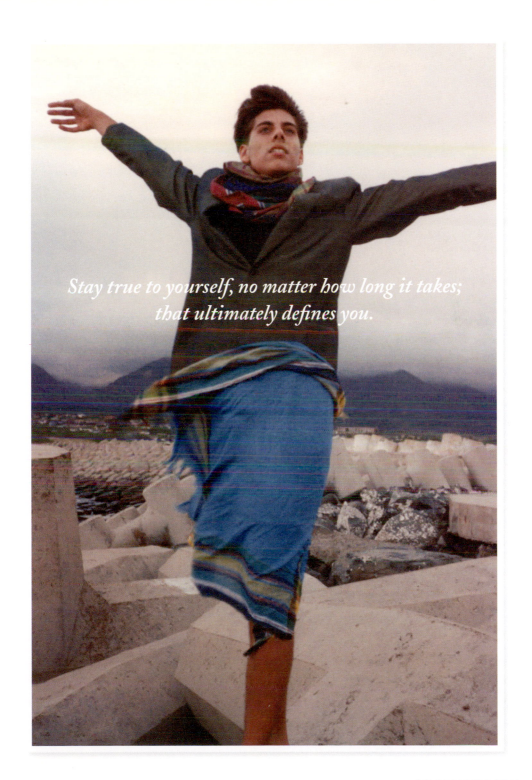

Stay true to yourself, no matter how long it takes; that ultimately defines you.

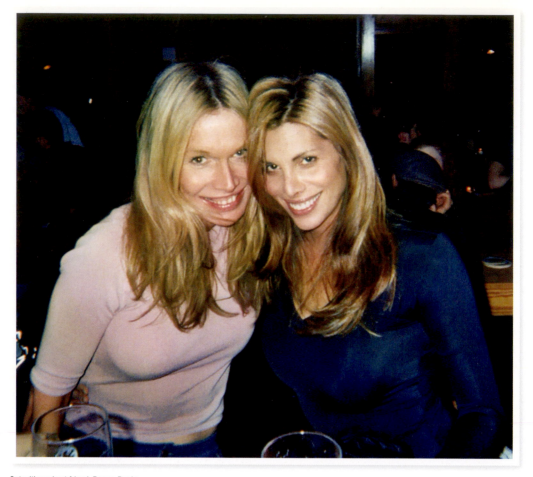

Out with my best friend, Danna Davis.

friend, Danna Davis. Once, on a flight, a sports team noticed that she was trans and started to berate her for the entire seven-hour flight. They were throwing paper wads at her the whole time; the flight seemed like it took forever, and when she finally came off the plane, she was mentally and physically exhausted and just wanted to get home. She got her bags, then looked up and saw the TSA agent that she still had to go through. She walked up to the agent, and it was a Latina woman with door-knocker earrings, the type of girl that would typically give "us girls" a hard time back then. She said to Danna, "Where are you coming from?" and Danna, almost in tears, said "Milan." The woman looked her up and down, and Danna thought, "Well, all right, here it comes." The woman said, "Well, how was your flight?" Danna, frustrated from her harrowing experience, said, "Do you want the truth?" The woman nodded her head and Danna said, "It sucked!" then told her everything that happened to her. The woman looked her up and down again, paused and said, "That ain't right, you can go ahead." Danna thanked her and started to walk away; after about ten steps, the woman said, "Ma'am!" Danna said, "Yes?" The woman said, "When you get to the end of the hall, turn around before you exit." So Danna turned at the very end of the hallway to see the customs agent with the entire team in a line, going through each and every bag, pocket, and suitcase, for hours to come. Danna turned back and exclaimed, "Gorgeous!" It's such a lesson in staying true to who you are, because moments like that truly transcend anything else.

As another example, just the other day, I had a comment on my Instagram from a girl I'd apparently met in the 1990s who said: "I met you at electrolysis and you gave me the stank face." What? I have never given *anyone* stank face! All I could say was "No, I didn't. I check myself, I don't allow myself to use whatever I'm going through to hurt anyone else." I'm not preaching here or trying to seem perfect, only to say this is about managing yourself, your body, your work, and your mind. It's all a choice for you, to either thrive or crumble.

Like all of us, I have had days when I've been so depressed I didn't want to get out of bed. What do you do about a funk like that? You allow yourself some TLC. You stay in bed, wallow in it, and allow yourself to experience it. But then, after a while, you start to think, "What can I do to change this situation?"

A lot of people see me on TV, and think I haven't had any struggles or problems. But let me tell you, living in New York City as a young trans performer, I had some truly rough times. Not only was there the trans thing, but also the woman thing. There are few of us on this earth who have had the ability to experience life as two different genders, and it has been interesting, to say the least. The way society treats you, the way men treat you, the list goes on. It's important for me to say that it's *not* okay to talk about women in negative ways. When I first started living as my authentic self, I was so excited to walk around New York City as the new me!

The very first day, I wore a fitted dress and was feeling so beautiful. As I crossed the street at 9th Street and Second Avenue, a truck drove by with three men in it, and one of them loudly yelled, "I want to lick your p###y!" Needless to say, I was horrified—and it changed the way I thought about how I presented myself to the world.

Anyway, as a young trans performer, there was no health insurance, no stability, and I would have to find other gigs all the time. So I went out and offered my talents to restaurants, retail shops, and other highly visible places. I did whatever I could to keep myself up, positive, and working, even when all the signs pointed in another direction.

We all know how hard it is to grow up in this crazy world, but you know what? It's so important to find the people who lift you up versus bring you down. These people are your chosen family—and they can be just as important to your survival as your birth family.

LIVE FOR YOURSELF

Twenty years ago, when my brother, Dylan, married his wife, Trudy, I was asked to be the best man at the wedding because he was my twin. I had just started to transition, and yet I had to go and be a good twin and give the best man's speech at the wedding. It was at that time that I realized I could not live for anyone else anymore, I had to live for myself. I love my brother and his wife, so I did what was necessary, but then I came home and promised myself I would never do that again. From that point on, I would live my life the way I wanted to live it. I think we all have experienced that moment

where you can either adapt yourself to meet the expectations of other people, or jump into the ring and live your life for you.

After my brother's wedding, I was so depressed. I came back home to my $600-a-month apartment at 14th Street and Ninth Avenue in New York City; mind you, this wasn't the glamorous 14th and Ninth Avenue of today, and it was definitely not a very safe place at the time. I had a bed and a kitchen where I stored my drag and paperwork, and that was literally all I had at the time. I remember looking at myself in the mirror, feeling so sad, when suddenly I saw a lilac aura around myself—and it was then that I knew I needed to live my life as a woman. I am still the same person I was before; I just needed to change the physical to match my heart and my mind.

I dove in and truly started the major steps that it took to live my life as a woman. I waited for about a year before I started to tell family, and finally one day I decided to tell my brother. Pensive but excited, I called up Trudy and Dylan and said, "I *have* to tell you about this!" Dylan said, "What? I didn't realize you felt this way!" Trudy, who studied sociology, explained to him what transgender meant, and Dylan got it. He accepted me for who I told him I really was, and has been a huge supporter ever since.

I felt so much happier when I started living as my authentic self. Brendan was a

It's so important to find the people who lift you up versus bring you down.

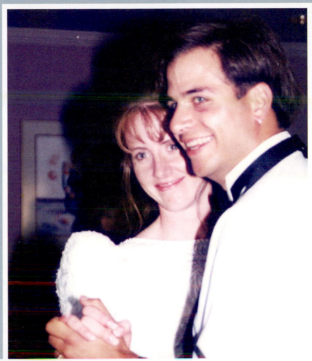

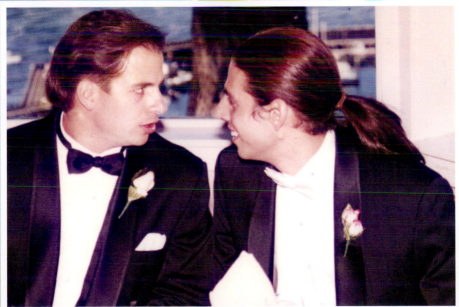

TOP: My brother, Dylan, and his lovely wife, Trudy.

BOTTOM: Me, on the right, serving as my brother's "best man."

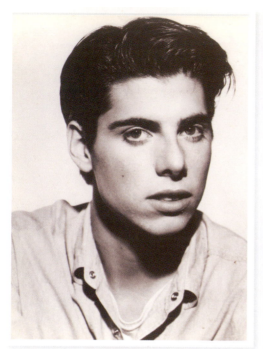

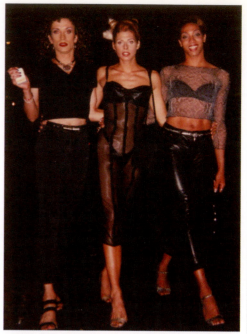

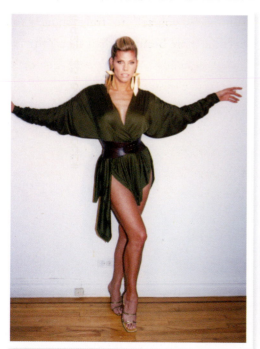

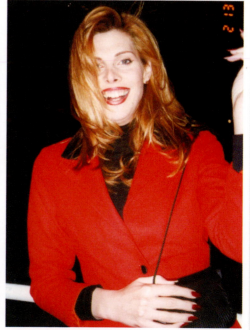

CLOCKWISE FROM LEFT: An early head shot; super-modeling with Shasta and Lina; Me, out and about in 1997; and playing model.

good, talented, and kind person, so I wasn't going to leave *him* behind. Today, I still feel the same as when I went by that name, because my mind was always female. Mentally, I feel exactly the same.

Two years after starting hormones, I packed up all of my old clothes and threw them into a bag. I took them down a New York City street in the middle of the night and threw them into the garbage. I woke up the next day, got ready for the airport, nervous but ready to do this. I dressed myself in a gorgeous pair of brown slacks with a demi pump and maroon sweater, and when I got to the airport, walked up to the ticket counter and nervously handed the agent my ticket, she said, "Thank you, ma'am, you can go on in." It was this magical moment that really started my new life, and I remember it like it was yesterday.

Think of your own "magic moment" of truth about who you are, in the deepest sense of the word. How are *you* living authentically—in a life that you designed specifically for your truest self? Where is your spiritual center, your "radiance spot"?

REDEFINE RADIANCE

Think of every woman you think of as beautiful. What stands out the most for you?

How has this become part of a narrow definition for yourself?

For me, true beauty is about grace, elegance, confidence, and inner beauty. It's a constantly moving target, too—one that's just as much about breaking the old paradigms that confine rather than empower us to redefine what beauty and radiance really mean—especially if that definition is different from anyone else's. It's about opening up the box and releasing all of the amazing colors of the rainbow, and not giving a second thought to what others will think, as long as we are happy and living the truth of our real selves.

You want to know what happens when you allow yourself to truly shine? You become more beautiful than ever. You radiate personality. You become magnetic, drawing the people, experiences, and fulfillment you most desire. All of us shine so much more brightly when we find and share our "radiance spot."

"But Candis—what if people don't like the real me?" you ask.

"Girl, what if they never actually *see* the real you?" I say. "How will they ever know who you are, or come to understand you like you understand yourself? Isn't that more important?"

We live in an exciting time, brought to us by a new generation who basically laugh in the face of established categories. They don't want to be defined by others, so they instead brought us fifty-eight categories of sexual identification on Facebook as well as phrases like "gender fluid." They are overwhelmingly in favor of LGBT rights, because they see them as human rights.

So, this is not just another beauty book, it's part of a much larger social movement—one based on breaking barriers and releasing the rigid definitions of the concept of beauty and who it is for. It's a call to action for all of us to wake up and celebrate our unique (and collective) beauty!

TAKE YOUR INNER BEAUTY OUTWARD

Remember Madonna's song, "Express Yourself"? (What can I say, I'm a child of the '80s!) The thing I will never forget is how it made me feel to know it was finally okay for all of us—gay, trans, queer, and straight—to express our true feelings. We didn't have to settle for second-best; we already deserved the best in life, as long as we expressed our true selves honestly. Women everywhere finally got the sense that they mattered *on their own*, without needing to wait for someone else to validate them.

Maybe you are just beginning to find your voice. Or you're tired of playing the game—and ready to reinvent yourself in a way that more authentically expresses your true personality. You're finally ready to spread your wings and soar as far as *you* can take yourself. How well you'll fly will depend on how strong you build your wings—and that's all about starting from the ground up.

This is all about how to train your mind and body, since changing your outlook is the biggest step forward you can ever take. The best place to begin is to ask yourself a few important questions: "Who am I?" "What defines my personality and beauty (both inner and outer)?" "What makes me shine?"

Your answers will ultimately lead you to discovering your "radiance spot"—the place deep inside your soul from where you can share that "radiant energy" of yours to create your own, unique style. One that's based on both the firm foundation of who you are now as well as the limitless heights of who you want to be in the future. One that rises above the "if onlys" to allow you, maybe for the first time ever, to shine your light into the Universe.

Let's celebrate the new, constantly changing and always growing YOU—because you have the right to express yourself as the best *you* possible!

INNER BEAUTY

What is inner beauty? It is often contrasted with outer beauty, found in the features (and movement) of the body. But where is inner beauty found? Its name suggests a hidden, unseen quality, but that's a misnomer. Inner beauty is seen because it radiates outward; it doesn't hide, but shines forth fearlessly. We all know people whom we would describe as having inner beauty, and we generally agree on who they are to us.

So, what are the criteria we use to designate someone as having inner beauty? What are some of the characteristics they have in common? When we think of some remarkable people we have known, several shared qualities begin to emerge.

Those with Inner Beauty (TWIB) have a lightness and purity of spirit; is this the thing that is beautiful? It exists regardless of how sullied the body's physical experiences. It persists when the person is burdened with the intensity of an extremely melancholic personality. There's an openness, an authenticity, a lack of deception. Such people are generally, although not always, of good cheer, though they are hardly Pollyanna-types.

TWIB are generous by nature. They're willing to help, even when it may be detrimental to their own interests (an annoying trait to their many friends). They're that first grader we all knew who undermined his own effort so that a needy friend could have the glory.

TWIB are courageous. Many are very strong in their individuality, in their principles. They frequently have the strength to stand up for what's right for themselves and for others—even in face of ridicule and scorn, not to mention the possibility (and sometimes the reality) of violence.

TWIB share many of these traits, but the essential ability necessary for real inner beauty is the ability to empathize in a real and meaningful way with others—to be able to understand the stresses and strains of another's life. Not merely an understanding of another's situation, but an imaginative shift into the other's emotional state to the degree of experiencing (a form of) that state.

The objects of TWIB's empathy frequently understand the insight they have, but are not offended. They are rather pleased, even grateful, for the understanding—grateful for being able to be oneself, free of judgment, around them. TWIB somehow have the ability, because of who they are, to create safe space for others—while at the same time, they create a feeling of deep caring and concern for well-being for all whom they encounter.

This is who our Candis is to us—TWIB extraordinaire, and someone we are so proud to call our daughter.

—Patricia Relles and
Gary McDanniel (my parents!)

MEET OUR BEAUTY TEAM

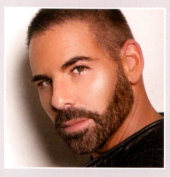

SCOTT BARNES is a celebrated makeup artist and innovator within the cosmetics industry. He has worked with world-renowned photographers, including Patrick Demarchelier, Francesco Scavullo, Gilles Bensimon, Tony Duran, Peter Lindbergh, and Annie Leibovitz. His work has graced the covers of such leading magazines as *Allure, Elle, Harper's Bazaar, Vanity Fair*, and *Rolling Stone*. Scott has also appeared on top national and regional television programs, such as *The Oprah Winfrey Show, Extra*, and *Access Hollywood*.

Although Scott has worked with a variety of Hollywood talent over the years—Kate Hudson, Nicole Richie, Mary J. Blige, Gwyneth Paltrow, and Céline Dion among them—it's his work with Jennifer Lopez that birthed the new monochromatic look featuring bronzed skin and pale lips. Described as "The Glow," this signature look became known as "lit from within" and helped launch Scott's best-selling beauty product, Body Bling Bronzer.

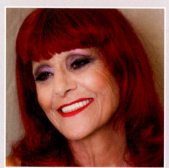

PATRICIA FIELD, a native Manhattanite, began her fashion career with the opening of her Greenwich Village boutique in 1966, at the age of twenty-four. For fifty years, her boutique has continued to be a globally well-known and respected fashion destination.

Patricia is especially famous for her Emmy Award–winning styling of HBO's *Sex and the City* from 1998 to 2004, for which she received critical acclaim and raised the standards in the world of television glamour through her costume design. A true pioneer, Patricia stimulated an entire fashion movement through the world in which high and low, old and new are mixed together with luxury design to create the "New High Fashion."

Patricia's impressive list of credits also includes *The Devil Wears Prada, Ugly Betty, Confessions of a Shopaholic*, and *Mother Goose Rock 'n' Rhyme* (for which she won another Emmy).

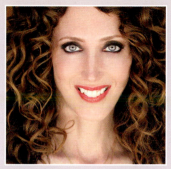

Costume designer and stylist **JENNIFER RADE'S** career encompasses everything from major red-carpet events and music videos to high-profile print and commercial advertising campaigns. She is a sought-after fashion commentator and style expert and has twice received the Costume Designer's Guild Award for Best Commercial Design. She has worked with photographers such as Patrick Demarchelier, Martin Schoeller, Norman Jean Roy, David LaChappelle, and Mario Testino, and her work has been featured in publications including *W*, *Vanity Fair*, *Marie Claire*, *GQ*, *Esquire*, and *Harper's Bazaar*.

How do you define beauty?

SCOTT BARNES:
"The very definition of beauty for me is individuality. It is always great to play up your best features and minimize the things you don't like as much. Everyone on this planet has a uniqueness and learning of what is inside of themselves, what they have to offer and how to bring it forward. That's the journey of self-discovery; embracing yourself bolsters confidence and strength of character, which I believe is the true essence of beauty."

PATRICIA FIELD:
"Beauty is both a subject and an object. Beauty boils down to a good and happy heart, a positive and confident attitude, and a helpfulness to others."

JENNIFER RADE:
"Confidence and self-acceptance."

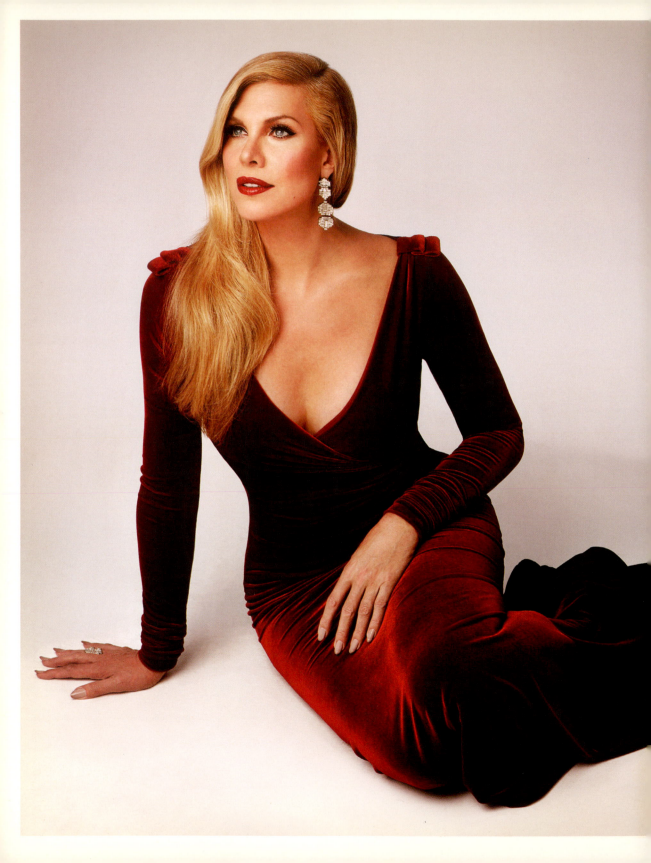

CHAPTER TWO:
AN INSPIRING
START

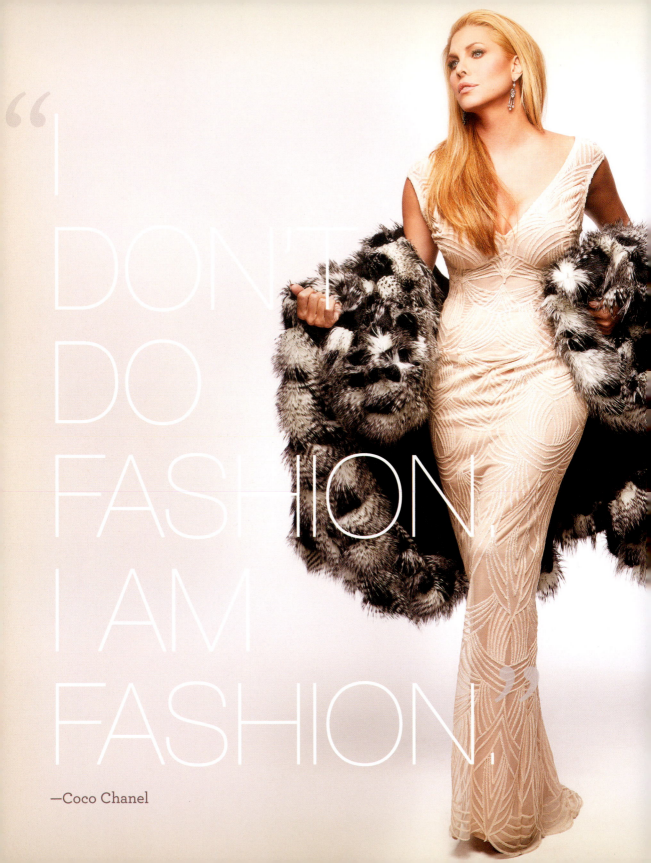

"I DON'T DO FASHION. I AM FASHION."

—Coco Chanel

et's face it—none of us would be where we are today without the inspiration of the other beautiful ones who came before us. For me, that means a whole host of lovelies, from old Hollywood icons like Cyd Charisse, Rita Hayworth, Grace Kelly, Marilyn Monroe, and both Hepburns (Audrey and Katharine), to the YouTube stars of today.

My own "style history" begins when I was about six years old. That's when I fell in love with Cyd Charisse's long, gorgeous, and graceful legs—which also inspired me to become a dancer. Cyd was the "It" girl of her time, and that was because she exuded a sexuality and level of confidence that transcended social norms of her time. She was amazingly gifted, yes—but also so lovely to look at. Who wouldn't want to be like her?

Then there was the classic loveliness of Grace Kelly, whose American good looks and carefree flip of blonde hair attracted a foreign prince. Elizabeth Taylor had those incredible violet eyes, while Marilyn Monroe showed the world that curves had a place in sexiness. From the exotic beauty of Sophia Loren and classic Jacqueline Kennedy Onassis to the sassy redheaded Ann-Margret and sultry Diana Ross, the Golden Age of Beauty continues to inspire women all around the world today—but it really had an impact on me as a kid.

It was hard for me to fully grasp the idea of how these memories would shape who I was as person, because after all, I was born a boy. Still, I was obsessed with the female persona. My twin brother, Dylan, was the epitome of masculine, and our cousins were male and female twins, so from early on, it was very confusing for me, because I couldn't figure out why I wasn't like my cousin Tonya. All I knew is that I wanted to be like her—and later on, like a plethora of other style icons.

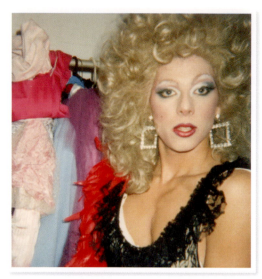 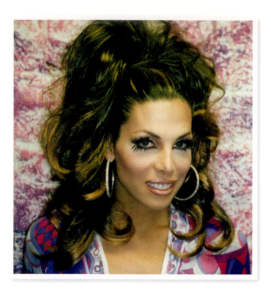

LEFT: My first time ever in drag.
RIGHT: A more "mod" look.

By my teen years, it was all about the creative expression of the inner self to the outer world. My fashion icons then were gender benders like Boy George (who could do all of his amazing makeup in less than fifteen minutes—by himself!), supermodels like Linda Evangelista, and Annie Lennox, who broke all kinds of barriers for deliciously androgynous women in the music industry. What I loved most about Annie was the structure of her amazing face, and her ability to constantly reinvent herself. Look at her old videos—she hardly ever appears the same way twice!

These icons were some of my guides along the path to becoming who I am today—and I still follow beauty, style, and power stars like Iman, RuPaul, and Meryl Streep, because they truly inspire me to become a better version of myself. Their grace, elegance, and inner beauty forces their outer beauty to shine more brightly— and makes them appealing to so many others. Don't you think they're all amazing?

THE MANY FACES OF BEAUTY

I was raised in a multicultural family (Italian, French, German, Scottish, Irish, and American Indian) in Hawaii, of all places, so I have always identified with many ideas of beauty. I thought that beauty was something you inherently possessed or something that you cultivated, but never something that was limited to a certain race, size, color, or gender. From my mom, I learned the power that a woman can possess (and also the misconstrued perceptions that come along with that power); from my father, I learned grace. And from my own experiences over time and geography, I learned that there are literally thousands of varieties out there in the human species. The need for acceptance is the one universal.

One of the biggest issues with young girls today is that so many of them do not see themselves in the pages of fashion and beauty magazines. The feminine ideal, at least in the United States, still seems to be aimed mostly at the blonde-haired, blue-eyed female—and because that describes me as well, I hope you get from this book that I am actually on your side. I think true beauty comes in so many wonderful sizes, colors, and shapes—like a big, beautiful garden full of all kinds of flowers. Wouldn't it be boring if we were all the same? Let's stop trying to fit into preconceived molds.

Think about the many ways you define beauty. Maybe you follow Michelle Phan, or Melanie Rodriguez, Patricia Bright, or Gigi Gorgeous on YouTube. It doesn't matter what their ethnicity might be, because we all have something to learn from each other. The key is to collect as many great ideas as you can, from as many sources as possible, in order to create a multifaceted, multiwonderful version of *you*.

FLASHBACK AND FASHION FORWARD

When I moved to New York City at age twenty-one, I had no idea what I was getting into. However, I don't regret a single day; I went there wanting to discover who I was as a person, and eventually as a woman. I didn't have two nickels to rub together, but back in the '90s, you could still live in Manhattan and be poor. I started working in the club scene and would go to all the thrift and vintage stores in town to look for fabulous finds. My friend Lina and I would scour all the monthly pages of *Vogue* and *Elle* to look for things we loved, and then we would go to the thrift stores and recreate those looks. It was amazing how accurate we could get—even sometimes finding looks in the same material! We learned the New York art of style, fashion, and accessories and all on a budget! I am a firm believer of using old and new together, wearing a fabulous jean jacket with a vintage top and jewelry, new shoes, and a vintage bag.

Back in my earlier days, lots of women wanted to be gender-bending, wearing the men's suit look like Diane Keaton (loved her in *Annie Hall*), Katharine Hepburn, and Greta Garbo. Some of us went the way of Madonna-inspired style and later moved on to grunge, while others of us preferred to

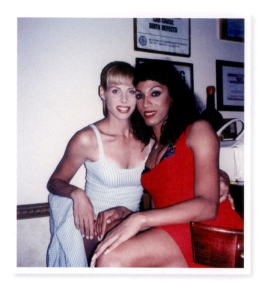

With my friend Lina.

style ourselves after classics like Coco Chanel, and Princess Diana, or transformative beauties like RuPaul. The '80s and '90s were times when a little bit of copy-cat behavior could go a long way in defining a strong look—and the fashion options were quite plentiful.

Today, there are more style and beauty options than ever before—with literally thousands of places online to buy whatever pieces you'd like, or can even dream up on your own for a custom look. It's literally a buyer's market, and if you have the money, you can invest in as much as you want or need.

But you want to know something? You don't need a Swiss bank account to look like a million bucks. If a piece speaks to you, try to figure out what it says about your personality, and then determine whether it's a good match. Whose look is this, really? If it's yours, roll with it. If it is just one that reminds you of someone else you admire, leave it for that person. You need to be your own "style whisperer" in order to generate the best looks for your personality. Living in New York taught me a lot about that concept, and now that I live in Los Angeles, I have found even more freedom in expressing myself through my own style. Your location will determine a lot of your style options, too. If you live in a colder climate, you'll be rocking sweaters and warmer clothes for a good part of the year. If you're a Southern peach, you'll be wearing much lighter, breezier looks. Out West, we girls tend to wear more of a sun-kissed look, where less is more. So, take your geography into consideration, and become a good reflection of the natural beauty around you. What are your local style icons wearing? How does that speak to you?

GIRL POWER

Beauty and fashion icons are just two parts of the whole equation. Female power is what I consider to be the final piece of the trifecta. When we think of beautiful women today, it's just as much about their

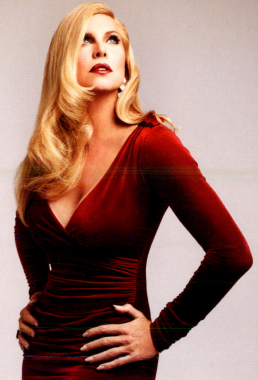
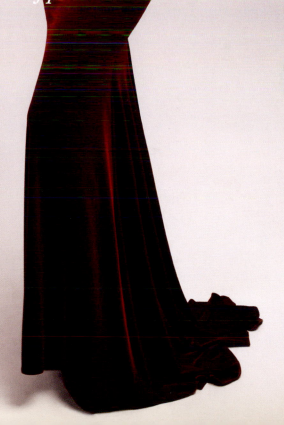

When we think of beautiful women today, it's just as much about their inner sense of power as it is about their outer looks.

inner sense of power as it is about their outer looks. When women like Cher, Jacqueline Kennedy Onassis, Diana Ross, and Madonna stepped up confidently in the '70s and '80s and started owning their power, something changed in them, both inside and out. Now we could see their inner selves more clearly than ever, and they were no longer the subservient, two-dimensional women of previous eras. With strong new role models like Beyoncé, Rihanna, Lady Gaga, Charlize Theron, Zhang Ziyi, Sofía Vergara, and Helen Mirren, we've definitely come a long way. However, take a closer look at the changing tides: Led by a more inclusive, accepting group of enlightened Millennials, we are now the ones who are defining who and what is truly female, and it's finally a much more encompassing definition than ever before.

I think of Tracey "Africa" Norman, the sixty-three-year-old former Clairol "Born Beautiful" model who, back in the '70s, hid the fact that she was the first black transgender model. She was on set for a shoot one day, and someone came in and whispered into the director's ear. The set was cleared, everyone was sent home, and she was fired. Finally, more than thirty years later, she received a call from Clairol—they wanted her to come back, to speak her truth to a new, much more accepting audience—and her inspiring video has since been seen by millions. The Nice'n Easy campaign said it loud and clear: "She's back, she's beautiful & she's her real self." The new campaign focuses on the "confidence that comes from embracing what makes you unique, and using natural color to express yourself freely." See? True beauty really is all about confidence—and sharing the light of your inner power.

PULLING TOGETHER YOUR BEST

Who are your beauty, fashion, and power icons, and how do they inspire and/or inform your own style? Can you easily separate them out, or are they pretty much running on a consistent theme?

Create a vision board or collage with all of them represented visually. Take pictures of things you like and keep them on your cell phone, or start a new Pinterest board as a visual shopping guide. Have fun with it—let your imagination enjoy the challenge of redefining your own style and beauty.

In case you haven't noticed by now, I'm a huge fan on finding a fun, unique style that's all your own and running with it—of course, with a few basic (and non-negotiable) rules:

PROPORTION: Most of us weren't born with the genes for a model body; you know, those girls who can wear a balloon and look fabulous. The rest of us have to live by other rules, and while rules were meant to be broken, you need to save your rule-breaking rebellion for color and pattern. Proportion is rarely an escapable thing for any of us.

COLOR: I'd like to think that most people can wear most colors, except for a few that just *don't* work. Mine is anything in neon peach, and most of the yellow family. I love color and I wear it all the time, but I also have my power colors; those are colors that when you wear them, you feel like a super-nova! We all have colors that just "work" for us, that we always look good in, and that we can rely on to carry a look. It really has a lot to do with hair color and skin tone, but finding your power colors will change your world! To learn how to find yours, go to my website: www.candiscayne.com.

PERSONALITY: Remember what I said about finding your style personality? That is one of the unshakeable truths in the power of personal style. It needs to be firmly established, but only for as long as you need to share an aspect of yourself, so it can evolve over time. As you age and grow, your personality does, too—and this can and should be expressed in your overall look. Honor the process of becoming yourself, because life is a miracle and every day is a new opportunity to shine.

Who is your beauty icon?

PATRICIA FIELD:
"Cleopatra."

SCOTT BARNES:
"There are so many and I've actually helped create a few, but if I were pressed to pick one I would have to say Raquel Welch. She's a beauty icon who also happens to be a good client and friend."

JENNIFER RADE:
"If you're looking at a celebrity as a beauty reference, chances are high that a professional artist did their makeup. So, then it's really the makeup artist that's the beauty icon! I think it's great to look at someone as inspiration for a great cat eye, smoky eye, red lip, or whatever it is you want to try—but ultimately beauty is about embracing yourself and working with what you have!"

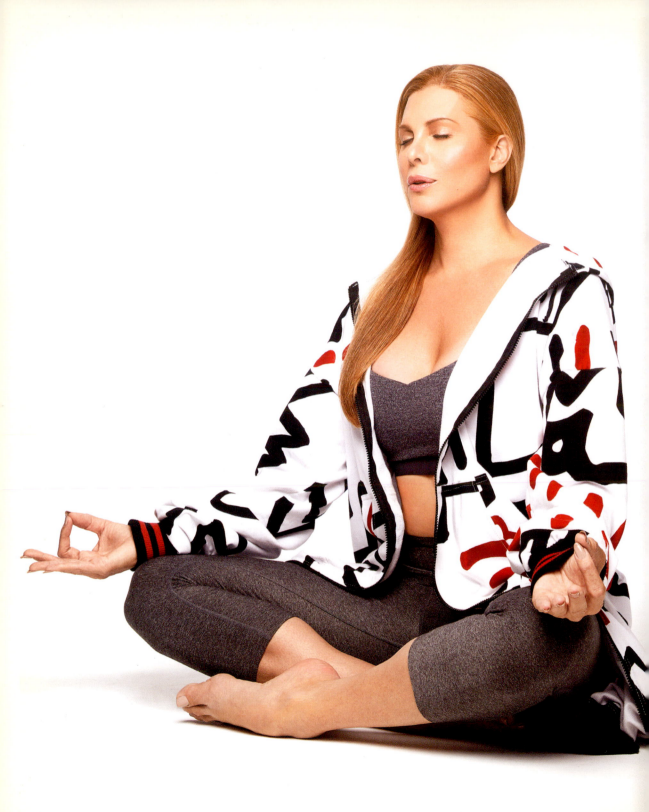

CHAPTER THREE:

INHABITING YOUR
TEMPLE

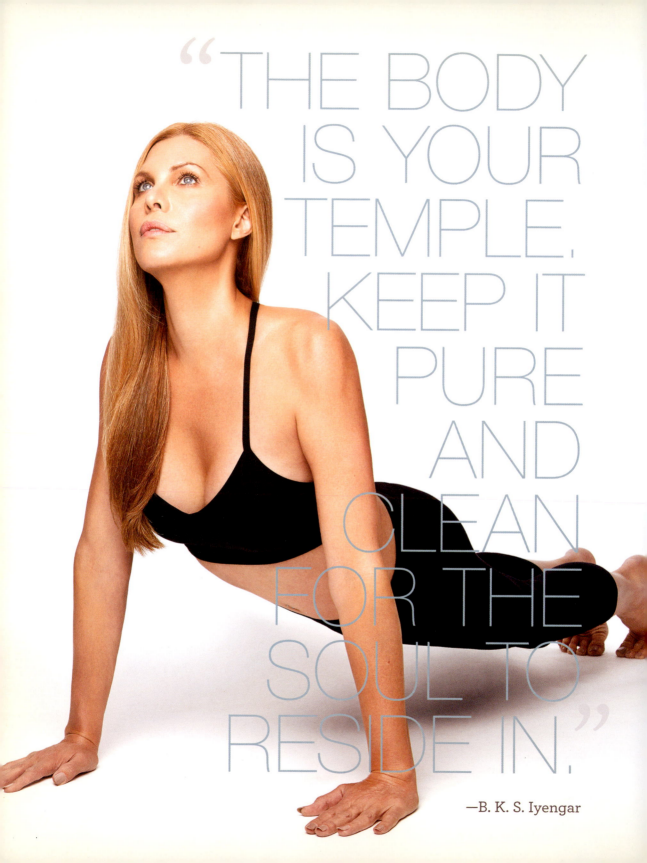

"THE BODY IS YOUR TEMPLE. KEEP IT PURE AND CLEAN FOR THE SOUL TO RESIDE IN."

—B. K. S. Iyengar

Many of us have a love/hate relationship with our body. It seems like no matter what we are born with, we always want something different. If we have curly hair, we'd rather have straight; if we're short, we'd prefer being taller. We're not all a size six—myself included. In my case, it was more about feeling like I was really a female in a male body, but for many of us, society and the media have taught us body-shaming from an early age—constantly pushing an unattainable image of perfection. But you know what? We have the power to change that, right here and now.

LOVING YOUR BODY

How and where do you start when you can't stand a lot of your body's "imperfections" or challenges? I've found that it's a lot like trying to fall asleep: You start at your feet, and work your way up your body until you've "relaxed" your thoughts about each and every square inch. Don't like your little toe? Start by telling it how grateful you are that it is part of your body, and how it helps you maintain balance when walking. Paint all of your toe nails a lovely color and appreciate each one as you are adorning them.

Speak positively to your body as you send it love and best wishes for the great day ahead. Be thankful for every single breath as you inhale and exhale. Life is good, and your body is an integral part of the whole human mosaic, right at this moment in time. You are supposed to be here, or you wouldn't be.

Body positivity is the key to being truly beautiful, inside and out. Expressing that through exercise, meditation, eating right, and a constant supply of self-respect is how you can build a better relationship with your own body. That's how you learn to listen to your body's "personal well-being" language. By hearing what your body needs—more rest, more water, less stress—you will learn how to best honor and support it. For me, this often means spending time close to nature—in my garden. Or taking a luxurious bath. Or doing yoga. Remember, the best way to stay beautiful is to keep your body happy and healthy!

There are so many good ways to honor your body, whether it's the one you were born with, or the one your inner being most sought to create. Let's practice a few.

IT ALL BEGINS WITH BREATH

One of the first things I learned as an actress is the importance of good breathing techniques. Did you know that most of us don't really know how to breathe correctly? If you're not doing it right, you can actually harm your body by depriving it of the vital oxygen it needs to regenerate every day. Holding your breath, or restricting it with tight clothing or daily stress, can result in less oxygen getting to your brain—and that can impact your ability to deal with even more stress, not to mention interfere with

getting a good night's sleep. No wonder you feel so tired all the time, right?

Lack of proper breath on a daily basis can also hurt your precious heart, because it can't possibly pump enough blood where it's needed without good support from the rest of your body. And it can prevent those fantastic endorphins from being able to spread some joy, too.

Breathing in and out through the nose, in a relaxed fashion and a comfortable pace is the very best way to breathe. You're less likely to inhale germs and allergens through your nose than through an open mouth.

One great way to practice breathing correctly is to lie flat on the floor, and put one hand over your diaphragm. If you can see your hand moving up and down, steadily and vertically, you are doing it the right way. This is also a great way to calm yourself if you are feeling stressed.

Another way to develop a healthier breathing regimen is to sit up straight in a chair, with your lower back against the back of the chair, and imagine you are a whale with a blowhole just above your tailbone. Breathe in calmly and deliberately through your nose, hold it for about five seconds, and then slowly release your breath out of your mouth while visualizing that it is moving down toward your tailbone "blowhole." This exercise helps you to calm your nerves before speaking, auditions, or

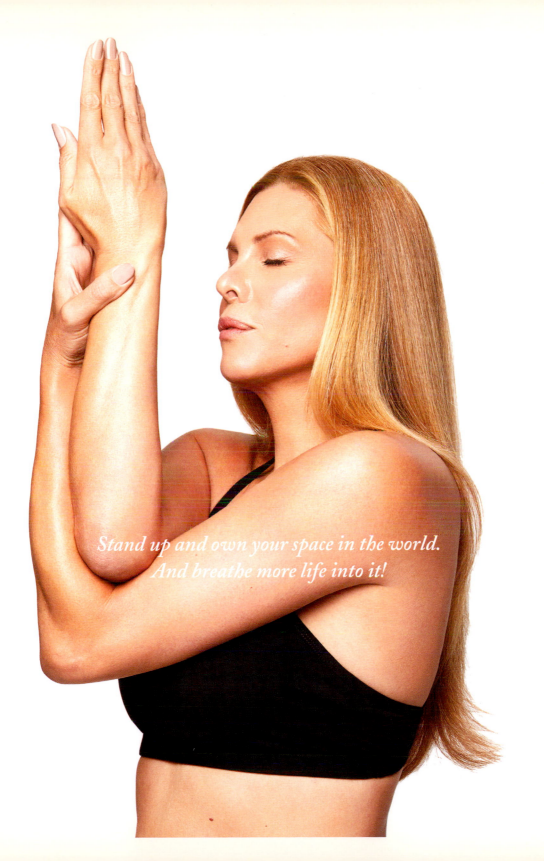

Stand up and own your space in the world.
And breathe more life into it!

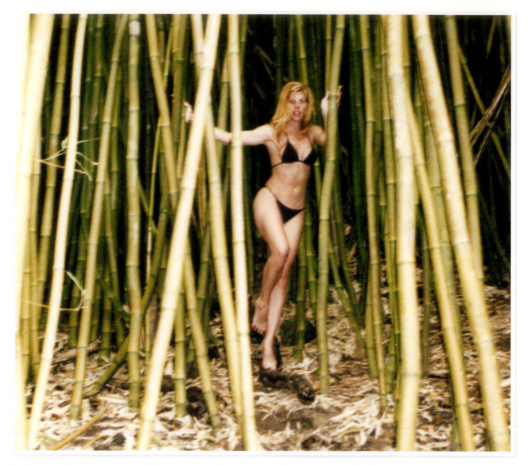

Visualize yourself in your happy place. This is me in Maui, at the Seven Sacred Pools bamboo forest in 2000.

any other kind of situation where you need to present your best self. I use it a lot, so I know it works!

Sitting (and walking) up straight is the best way to ensure that all that wonderful oxygen is flowing properly throughout your body. How many of us have terrible posture, the result of years of being told to make ourselves "smaller"? Stand up and own your space in the world. And breathe more life into it!

FINDING YOUR HAPPY PLACE

Visualization is another great way to help control your stress level in order to keep your body happy and healthy. Where are you your happiest, most calm, most peaceful, gorgeous self? Is it at the beach, with the waves rolling in just before a lovely sunset?

Or in the mountains, watching the morning mist give rise to the sun? Maybe it's simply in a comfortable room of your home, sitting by a window or fireplace—or, if you're like me, in your garden. Wherever it is, make a mental note of it, because it will be the best instant medicine you can give yourself in a moment of distress. Life is beautiful, but it also throws us a few curveballs at times to keep it all interesting. How we handle each setback is what makes us stronger, so you need to create a portable, visual "medicine chest" that you can use whenever and wherever you need it. Your body will thank you

MOVE IT, ALREADY!

Like any good machine, your body needs motion in order to keep working—especially if you have more of an office- or desk-bound life during the daytime. It is so important to get on some sort of workout regimen, even if it's simply walking three times a week. It's not only good for your body, but for your mind as well.

I had formal training as a dancer, so I love to dance, even if it's just for myself. Put on some music and get moving! It's

Remember, the best way to stay beautiful is to keep your body happy and healthy!

every time you use these tools to find your happy place, and return to a state of peace and well-being.

Our society is so Type A, so fueled by caffeine and meds many of us don't even need. Everything we need to survive is literally in the palms of our hands, and we can summon our own bodies to serve us in just about any way we need to, at any moment. Think about situations where people can suddenly do very heroic things to help their loved ones in an emergency situation—can you even imagine? And yet, it is possible. The human body is truly an amazing machine.

amazing what a few great songs can do for your mentality; in just a few dance moves, you can quickly coax your body out of the blues. Whenever my friend Danna comes to visit, we buy three bottles of wine, put on some records, and dance. I love it! We have a disco party.

Workout is key for just feeling good—and not just on the outside, but on the inside, too. For me, to truly feel at my personal best, I work out four or five days a week—early, for an hour, and the rest of the day I don't even think about it (unless I'm sore!). I give myself time off (for good behavior) on the weekends. After doing it for a bit, I promise you it will turn into a fun thing.

I do boot camp, and before that I used to do gym cardio, and before that it was dance class. No matter what your body type is, it's great to just be active. That doesn't mean hardcore stuff, but just something that gets you up and moving. If you decide to go for a great walk around your neighborhood at least three days a week, you'll carry yourself differently, feel stronger, and be in a better mental state.

Some people need structured meditation; I've never been able to do that. I'm a dancer with too much energy, so I tend to meditate when I am doing things like gardening, tending and nurturing those plants, and tuning out the rest of the world. In the garden, I can breathe. Dance class does that for me as well. Being completely present, yet free at the same time, to forget whatever else is going on; to delve so deeply it becomes a meditative state. Working out regularly has gotten me to the point where I can exercise and have fun, right there in the moment. That's what meditation is essentially—calming your mind and allowing your brain to get a break.

Lately, I've been getting into Vinyasa yoga once a day as a more meditative practice, and it has completely changed my outlook. It's amazing, because while true beauty is all about accepting yourself as

you already are, yoga is all about accepting each moment, on its own terms. And it's not too hard; you just do a series of sequences that open up your flow, help ease back pain, and help you achieve better breathing, coordination, and alignment in your spine and back. Breath is coordinated with movements, as you flow from one pose to the next.

You can always sign up for a class, or work with a trainer, to become a better friend to your body. The level of commitment is entirely up to you—just know that you don't need to make it complicated in order to get decent results, especially if you are simply exercising for daily well-being. Many women psych themselves out and feel too overwhelmed by their lives to even consider committing to a formal exercise regimen—and that's one reason why we have such a high obesity rate. Let's buck that trend by keeping it simple and achievable.

DIET TRIPS

One exercise we can all do less of is the walk from the sofa to the refrigerator. I know it's easier said than done, but if we take the one small step of drinking more water every day, our stomachs will be fuller and we'll crave less of the junk foods out there. Getting enough water is the single most important dietary requirement to follow. If you think it's too boring on its own, squeeze a whole piece of citrus in there, or even some watermelon, and I promise it'll be refreshing. Stay away from sugary drinks and sodas, because not only will they make you put on weight, they'll also wreak havoc on your teeth and gums over time. I, for one, would rather save my sugar for ice cream than a soda any day. I drink a lot of water so much that I don't enjoy life. I try to eat well and make food as much as I can from scratch, so I can occasionally indulge in certain guilty pleasures. I try to eat organic, mostly because I want to know where my food comes from, who made it, and how authentic it really is. I try to get whole foods and create dishes with those ingredients. You don't have to be a chef; just have a few good cookbooks around and try some

GLAM ON THE GO

To curb cravings, I pack fresh fruit, vegetables, and organic snacks—and tons of water. It's the best way to stay healthy and energized all day long. Also, when traveling, always take a small neck pillow with you. Wrap it around the handle of your suitcase and use it whenever you need it. Just getting a fifteen-minute nap can reenergize your body, making for much smoother sailing.

every day, and it helps me to stay healthy, energized, and improves my skin. There are so many benefits waiting for you in at least six to eight glasses of water per day.

We don't all need to be on an insanely restrictive diet to be healthy and beautiful. It's all about training your mind and body to respond to your own positive feelings about yourself. And that starts by looking at your relationship with food.

I absolutely love food of all kinds. I love everything about it, so like many women, I have to keep myself in check—but not

things. If you're craving mac and cheese, learn how simple and how much better it is if you make it yourself. I know, you're saying, "How could I possibly do that when my time is already so limited?" But if you start to learn about what goes in your body and how to make it, you'll get addicted to experimenting with cooking deliciously healthy meals.

I love pasta, but switch it up by using quinoa with a tomato sauce sweetened with two whole carrots; it's not hard to make healthy changes like that when you're cooking at home.

French fries are by far my guiltiest pleasure. What can we do about such evil cravings? Here's how I handle it: once or twice a week, I say F@$#K it and get whatever I want. To me, that's still being healthy, as long as it's kept in moderation. If you can't control yourself, then don't take the risk. Remove all of those temptations from your kitchen, and stock it with healthier options only. At least until you can get a handle on it. Then follow the simple rule: eat less, move more.

BOOK SOME "YOU" TIME

Every temple requires some down time, and your body is no different. Why do we push ourselves so hard, and then wonder why our bodies are falling apart at younger and younger ages than in the past?

A huge part of being good to yourself is accepting that your body needs relaxation in order to regenerate cells, from your skin to your brain. That means at least eight hours of sleep every single night—and frequent periods of unplugging from the rat race of life. By that, I mean turning off your computer or phone, and truly engaging in an activity that relaxes you and makes you feel more positive. Not a walk in which you gossip to your best friend on your cell

about who did what to whom last night, but a quiet, peaceful time in which you can disconnect mentally from all that is happening around you, and simply be.

For a lot of us, this is a challenge to accomplish on our own. Honey, that's why God invented spas and massages. Finding a good spa is like finding a good doctor—you'll need to ask around, and check out reviews online. You can even get a massage in the comfort of your own home. Now it's easier than ever before with some great, at-your-fingertip tools like the apps Soothe and Zeel, which allow you to book an in-home massage session with a licensed therapist. Using Soothe is perfect for my crazy busy schedule. If I can do find time for it, you can, too. And guess what? It can often be less expensive than an in-studio massage session—and more comfortable for you, being in your natural surroundings.

Carving out some "you" time, at least once a week, can be a challenge for many of us—but don't use time as an excuse not to try. You and your gorgeous body are so worth it.

CELEBRATE, DON'T BERATE

I had to physically become my own temple to have peace of mind and live in my authentic skin, as my true self. Surgeries were part of that for me; it's also been about being healthy and fit, and feeling good about myself and my body. I love a glass of wine at the end of the day; I try not to over-indulge, but to just give myself moments. Transitioning is a daunting task—the surgery, hormones, electrolysis. You have to do it soundly, safely, and for the right reasons. I would never have a surgery because I thought I wasn't good enough the way I am; I only wanted to enhance who I was already.

It's good to realize that who you are is an incredible, amazing thing and it should be celebrated. You don't have to kill your spirit working out like crazy or dieting to an extreme where you are not happy. Seek out the regimen that works best for you. The most important thing you can do to honor the temple of your body is to love it unconditionally—the way you already do for your best friends. I make the time for things in my life that bring me joy—like gardening, shopping, playing volleyball, or spending time with friends and my dogs. You were probably expecting to get lots of exercise moves in this chapter, but you know what? The most important thing in life is a healthy mind, body, and soul. I've been through a lot and I know how hard it is to accomplish even simple things when you're not in the right space to do them, so it's so important to learn to listen to yourself and deliver whatever you most need. If you're not getting enough of that inner happiness that makes you shine, make it happen today. Celebrate who you know yourself to be—and stop all that negative self-talk. The power to make yourself feel better lies within you!

What's something you can do to feel better about yourself?

JENNIFER RADE:
"Call a friend who makes you laugh. Laughter makes everyone feel better. Also, there is beauty in everyone. It could be a pretty smile, great shoulders, great skin, a quick wit. It's important to remind yourself what's beautiful and unique about you."

SCOTT BARNES:
"Love yourself. I have to quote my favorite poem, 'Desiderata,' by Max Ehrmann, which encapsulates this sentiment: 'Beyond a wholesome discipline, be gentle with yourself. You are a child of the universe, no less than the trees and the stars, you have a right to be here.' This is a very powerful mantra."

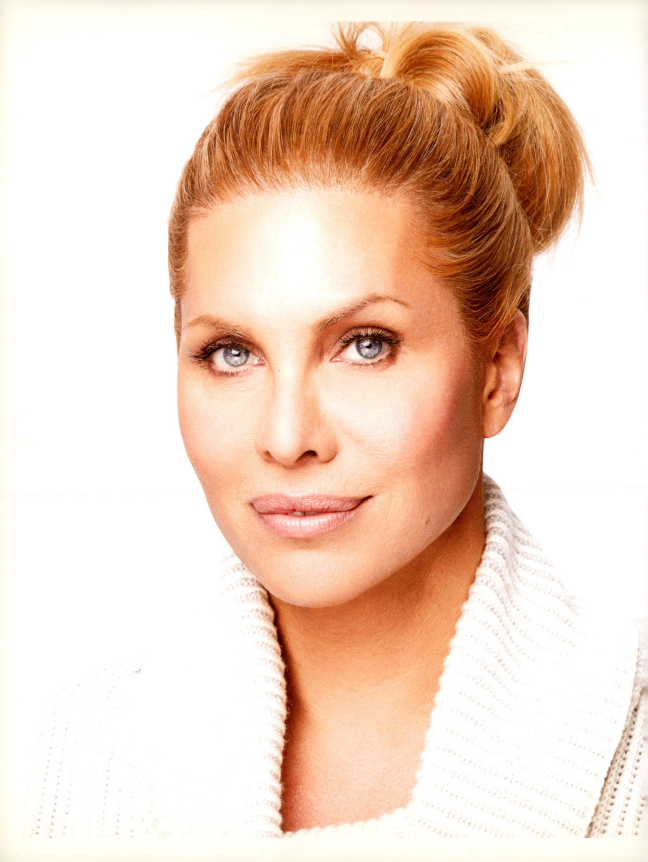

CHAPTER FOUR:

A PRETTY
PALETTE

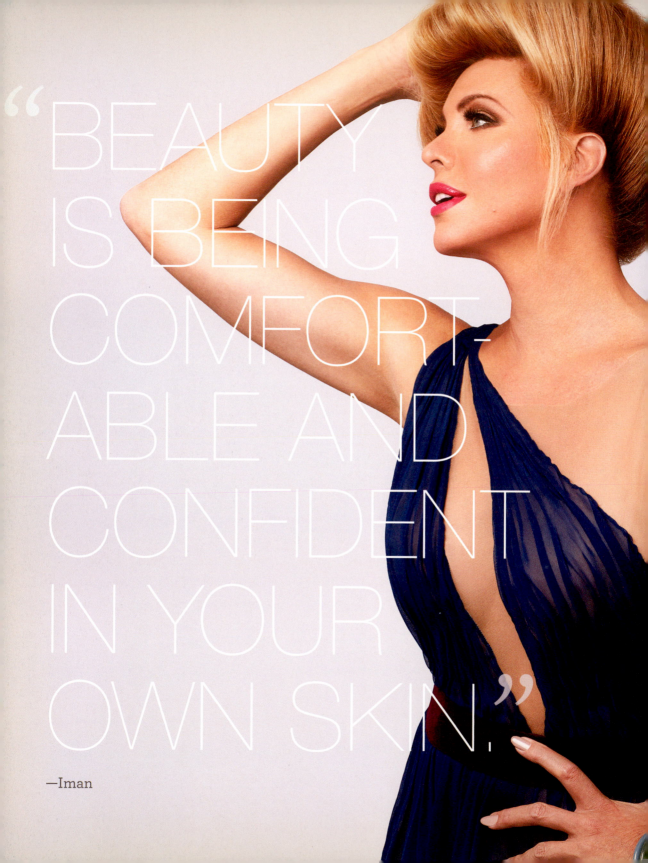

"BEAUTY IS BEING COMFORT-ABLE AND CONFIDENT IN YOUR OWN SKIN."

—Iman

Radiant beauty is built upon a blank canvas—a clear skin palette, kept clean with a solid skincare routine, and a strong, smooth foundation that supports loveliness across the entire skin-type spectrum. Simply put, there's nothing more beautiful than your own gorgeous, natural skin, with its perfect imperfections that make you the wonderful you that you are right now.

When you think about it, your skin is kind of like nature's miracle material—it can withstand so much stretching, blemishing, and abuse from chemicals, and yet it's always regenerating and healing itself in the process. That's pretty amazing—and why it's so important to clean, nourish, and protect your "outer shell" as much as possible. Impurities hit your face and skin every single day; it acts as an environmental windshield. Everything that hits your skin affects it. That's why you need to really invest in some great skin-care products, first and foremost, along with the usual regimen of keeping hydrated.

I know I've talked about the importance of water already but it's worth repeating when we're talking about improving your skin. Water is the source of life. Our bodies are made up of about 65 percent water, and so much out there totally depletes it: soda, coffee, stress, heat, the environment. Switching even one cup of coffee a day for water will improve the look and feel of your skin. The older I get, the better my skin looks in a lot of ways, and drinking plenty of water has made all the difference.

PROPER FACE-WASHING

Of course, water isn't just for drinking—it's also for cleaning your outer shell. With all of the impurities out there, you need to learn how to wash your face properly, preferably with a few splashes of refreshingly cold water afterward.

You need a gentle cleanser to clean pores without blocking them up, which is what leads to pimples. Here's the process:

• First, remove your makeup with an oil-based remover (or wipes).
• Next, use a gentle cleanser based on your skin type (Clinique or Kiehl's are highly recommended). Make sure you spread it all over your face, to the hairline.
• Rinse with lukewarm or even cold water.
• Lightly pat with a towel (never rub!).

For a "spa-like extra," cool off from a long day with water-soluble vegetables like fresh cucumbers on your eyes; these will also help you get rid of any "excess baggage" you might be carrying under your eyes, and will help you feel fresh and hydrated throughout the night.

Exfoliation is critical to a good skin-care routine. I use supergentle exfoliants at home, two to three times per week to cleanse myself of all of the Los Angeles smog. If you live in a larger city, you should do the same. Wash and exfoliate to clear off dead skin and the big-city nasties, then do a swatch of either rosewater or glycerin spray. Follow with a moisturizer that is calibrated to meet the needs of your skin. Marilyn Monroe used an almond oil product called Aura Glow back in the day to give her skin a natural softness and shine, and that product is still available today at the Heritage Store (www.heritagestore.com).

Choose carefully based on your skin type, because if you use the wrong products, it will make your skin break out, and we don't want to go backward in this process. For instance, heavier oils may be great for those with dry skin, but awful for those with oily or combination skin. If you aren't sure what your skin type is, consult with a professional dermatologist or cosmetologist. It's worth it to get a proper evaluation of your skin's specific needs, so that you don't waste money on products that just don't do what they're supposed to do for you.

SUN-KISSED (AND LOVED)

Growing up in Hawaii and now living in California, being a sun worshipper is kind of in my DNA. Still, I take care to protect myself from harmful rays, and I spray-tan for special events rather than submitting my body to the damage that occurs from laying out in the sun all day to achieve a bronze glow. I get that many still prefer to bake in the sun to give your skin more color;

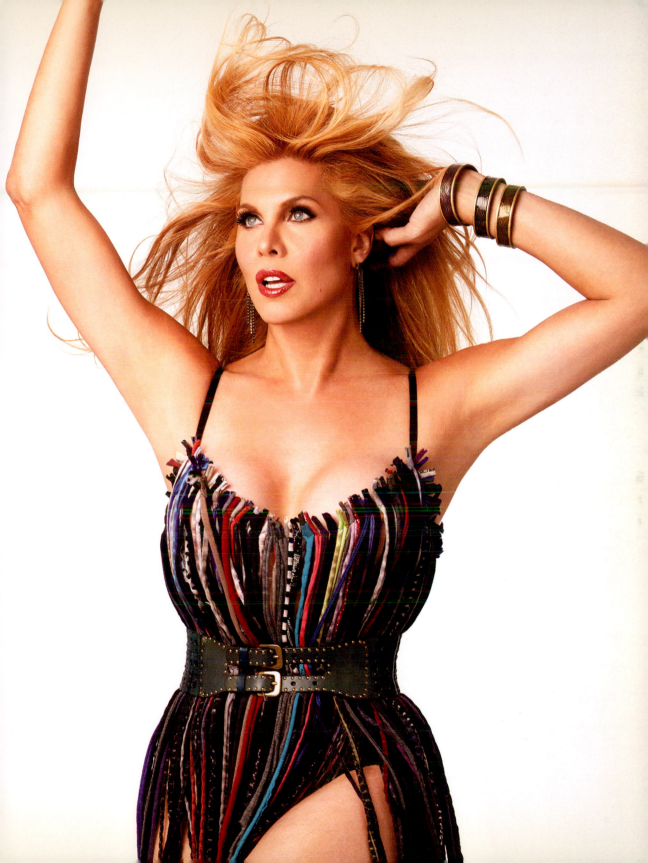

just make sure you're using a product that's at least SPF 45 to avoid potential threats from too much sun exposure like premature aging and skin cancer later on. There are so many fantastic (and harmless!) bronzers and plant-based self-tanning products available, you really should take advantage of these wonderful options to keep your skin in optimum shape. No one wants their skin to look like those leather-faced cowboys in the old Hollywood westerns. Exfoliate first, so your tan stays smooth and lovely for as long as possible.

The best way to get a spray-tan is to go to a professional. This way, you can make sure it is done evenly and thoroughly, so you don't go outside looking like a spotted leopard. Check reviews online, or better yet, get a good referral before you go. It may cost a little bit more, but a smooth, even look will be worth it.

If you are set on tanning naturally, limit the time you spend in the sun to two hours or less, take frequent breaks, and always keep some aloe vera and cold cream on hand, in case you do burn. Aloe works wonders—it's gentle on your skin and is inexpensive, to boot.

Finally, remember that you'll need to move to a darker shade of foundation for your summer look. Or just use a good bronzer and a nice kabuki brush to bring your sunny side out.

PERFECTING IMPERFECTIONS

What about the more permanent kinds of "imperfections"? Honey, we all have things we hate about our skin, but some things we just need to learn how to work with in order to turn them around:

MOLES, BIRTHMARKS, AND BEAUTY MARKS: One of my favorite memes is one that reads, "Honor your ancestors, for you are the result of a thousand loves." That means your natural marks—all of them—have been passed down to you from all of the people on your family tree. There are also those who believe that they are mystical marks from past lives. Whatever they are and wherever they came from, you can easily play them up by minimizing your makeup around them, or transform them with a lovely accent color, body jewelry, or even a small henna or tattoo. Marilyn Monroe and Cindy Crawford made their beauty marks a brand statement, and you can, too, by just adding a little dark pencil to make it stand out.

FRECKLES: Typically, it's the gingers who have a lot of freckles. Fortunately, a light base or foundation, dusted with peach-colored blush or a light bronzer for highlights, can totally illuminate your face and make your freckles seem like constellations. Use a matching lip gloss to keep it all as naturally gorgeous as possible. With freckles, you were born adorned, so play it light on the face and use nail and clothing colors to add a splash of fun.

HAIR: Okay, none of us appreciate facial hair, especially those of us who are trans and had to face the idea of going through puberty with testosterone. Should you shave it, use a hair removal cream, or have it professionally removed? My opinion is that professional removal works best and longest, while shaving is the worst, because it will lead to faster-growing hair and will come in coarser over time. You can pluck an occasional hair, but if it keeps coming back it needs to be treated. That means even if you're not a male from birth, you're going to see a five-o'clock shadow like one over time. Avoid the drama by going with removal cream at home, or a professionally done electrolysis every other month.

ECZEMA: For those who suffer from eczema, the struggle is real. You may feel that any makeup is irritating enough to cause a flare, but don't worry—there are still some good options. First off, go totally fragrance-free and hypoallergenic, and stick with products that don't contain lanolin. Buy fresh, new cosmetics on a

quarterly basis, because many makeups contain germ-breeding preservatives. Along the same lines, I recommend applying cream makeup with sponges or your own, clean fingers versus brushes. For powder foundations and eye makeup, you can use well-made brushes (the cheaper ones leave brush hairs all over your face). Keep it as light and naturally gorgeous as possible!

PIMPLES: The best way to avoid pimples is to drink plenty of water and keep your pores clear and open as much as possible, which means limiting makeup or going with lighter, mineral-based powders. If you still have issues, see a dermatologist and perhaps get prescription-level help; often, a simple round of antibiotics can get your skin clear again in a short period of time. You can also try to find out whether you have any allergies, because many times those can be the culprits. For temporary blemishes, try using a good astringent and some cover stick until it passes. I've never tried the *Big Fat Greek Wedding* Windex method, but it makes sense that any product with alcohol in it, even hand sanitizer, would be of assistance. Just don't make the situation worse by trying anything too harsh for skin. (Hint: If it burns, it's probably not the best thing to be using.)

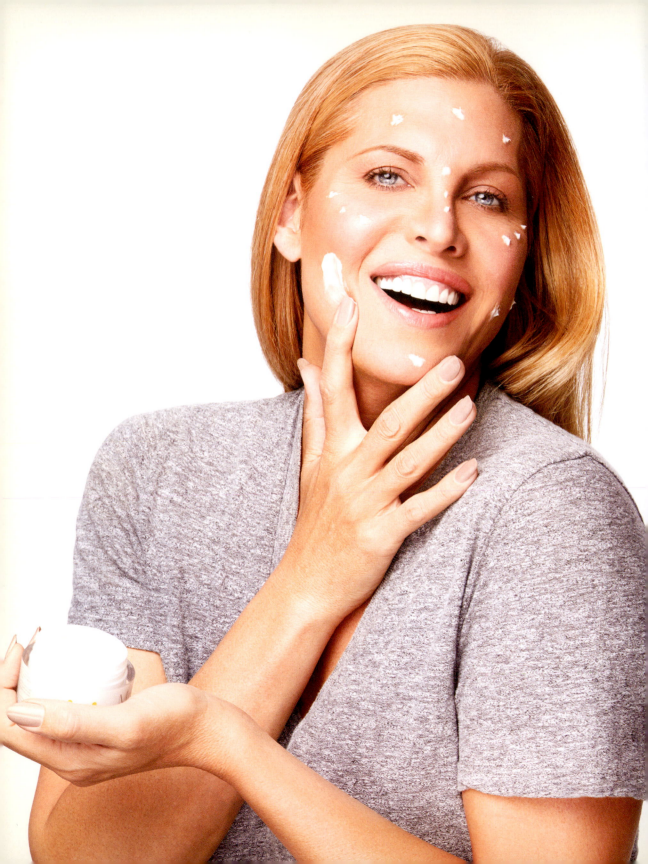

DISCOLORATION: The best way to even out blotchy or discolored patches of skin is to color-match as closely as possible, then apply slightly more makeup to the affected area and less everywhere else. Concealers and dermatologist-developed products such as Physicians Formula can also help even things out, and restore you to whole-

AGING: You're getting older, and wiser, so remember the adage "less is more." Too much makeup can make you look older if it's not applied right. Creams in particular can find their way into your nooks and crannies faster than you can say "granny panties." Use a soft powder foundation with a light blush, and play up your eyes

GLAM ON THE GO

To do a "cucumber cool-down" at home, keep a sleep mask in your freezer and fresh cucumbers in your fridge. Simply slice off two pieces of fresh cucumber (one for each eye), and then put the cold sleep mask over them to cover your eyes. Just a ten-minute refresh will help get rid of bags under your eyes, and keep you looking fresh and awake all day long. You can also heat up the sleep mask in the microwave if you prefer a warm treatment. This is a supereasy—and supercheap—home spa session!

Want some good advice for dealing with blemishes while on the road? If one pops up when you're traveling, put some toothpaste on it and it will be way less noticeable by the next morning.

some perfection. I like to apply concealer with a wet brush and powder, because it goes on smoothly and beautifully. Cream sticks, especially for covering large areas, create too much of a patchy, chalky look, so avoid those for anything other than undereye action. During the day, I apply a little bit of light-tinted moisturizer that evens everything out. I tend to get a little flushed, so I like to have that light amount of extra coverage.

and lips because they tell your real story of inner youth. But remember, you should do what feels right for you! Just learn the proper steps to make it look great.

"SKINCLUSIVE" TIPS

I have some tips for every woman—starting with my own regimen. I'm kind of addicted to Kiehl's products. I really like their Midnight Recovery Cream and their Ultra Facial Cream Moisturizer, and I use those daily to keep my skin in its best form, followed by Pond's makeup remover at the end of the day.

How about you? Let's take a closer look at recommended regimens for each of the five main skin types:

NORMAL: Oh, lucky girls! For you, it's all about keeping it clean and clear. You tend to look fabulous whether or not you're

spray on and blend some rosewater and glycerin oil for a light finish overnight. You really don't need heavy creams at night, because that's when your body's natural oils come out to play. Let nature take care of itself, darling.

OILY: A good glow is amazing, but does your face shine a little too much—like you've been running a marathon in the desert? Or like you've bathed in bacon grease? Hush, no worries. Wash twice daily with warm water and acne-control

Remember, you should do what feels right for you!
Just learn the proper steps to make it look great.

wearing makeup, so dress your face up or down to your heart's content. Stick with a good line of skin-care products for as long as it works for you, and be grateful for your good fortune.

DRY: Flaky or dry skin is usually the result of environmental damage, whether it's from external things like weather or product choices leading to contact dermatitis. You could be allergic to the soaps or cleansers you're using, so try switching to a glycerin-based soap or gentle daily exfoliator with refreshing citrus notes to make your face feel fresh and clean all day long. Repeat the same process at night, and then

products that help inhibit the amount of oil blocking your pores. Don't scrub too hard, because that will only inspire more oils to spring forth. Witch hazel with a drop or two of lemon juice, or a mint-based herbal toner, can also work wonders. Apply some loose powder as a boost a few times throughout the day to wipe off that shine without ruining your look.

COMBINATION: So, you've got a little bit of everything going on, depending on where we're looking at your face? Sounds like combo skin. Most often, it's your T-zone (across your nose) that is oily, but you're dry around the forehead, cheeks,

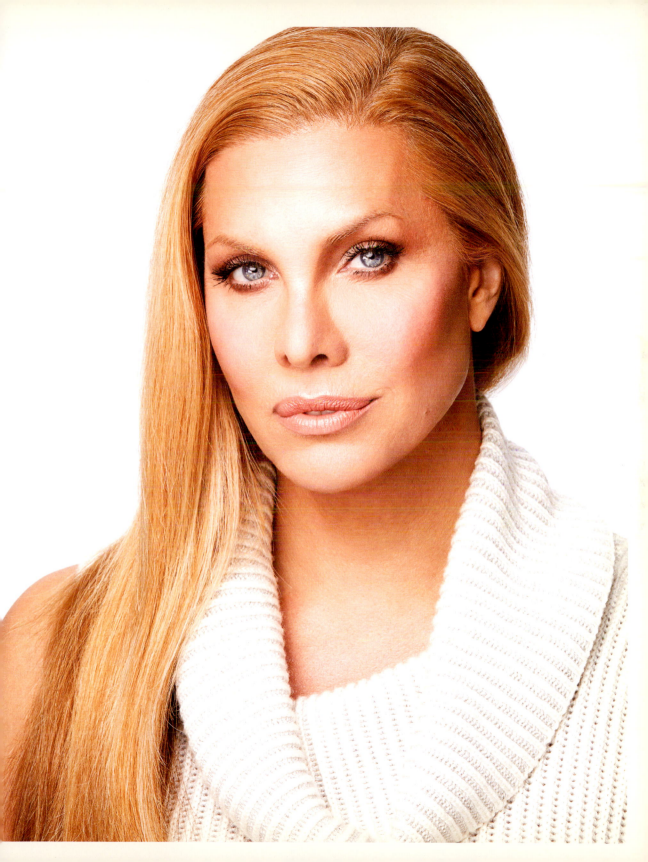

and chin. This is caused by different pore sizes, so you'll benefit from a good product (like Clinique) that can adapt to your skin's many needs.

SENSITIVE: Does your skin get easily irritated, like a bad mother-in-law? Is it prone to instant breakouts that come and go literally overnight? If so, you may have sensitive skin, and that will likely require some dermatologist-recommended products, or you can simply try staying with natural products such as mineral makeup.

BREAK UP OR MAKEUP?

The amazing Alicia Keys has been at the forefront of the #NoMakeup movement, a call to women to celebrate their inner beauty by skipping makeup altogether. It's an empowering concept, isn't it? How often do you go without makeup, and how does it make you feel? Are you afraid to let anyone ever see you without makeup, and if so, why? When I go out into the world, I never wear full makeup; I just use a self-tanner and a little hint of bronzer for a no makeup/ makeup look. This can easily be enhanced or made more dramatic for an evening look. For me, it was important to get to a point

where I didn't have to wear makeup, to feel even more authentically female. I only use makeup to enhance who I am, not change who I am—and that's what you should use as your true foundation as well. It's amazing how freeing it can feel to show the world your true face.

TRANSFORMING TREATMENTS

So, confession time: when it comes to skin and beauty, I am not necessarily a "purist." By that I mean, I think there are some real benefits to be had from treatments like Botox, hair removal, laser therapy, and even certain surgeries, as long as they enhance without damaging. Obviously, I've had my own surgeries and special treatments in order to live more fully as a woman, and that's how I've chosen to achieve an overall glow. For me, it's been a long, sweet journey to womanly beauty—and one that I totally respect by honoring my skin with a good maintenance regimen. Aging is one thing, but how you feel while you're aging is what makes the difference.

Particularly because of my journey, I'm often asked about my philosophy of what good skin care can do emotionally as part of a woman's self-care program. It makes a world of difference—it can be the determining factor in a woman's confidence level in going out, and in sharing who she really is with others. I go to a place called Prolase Laser Clinic (to my girl, Mrs. Tancura) for my maintenance with facials and hair removal. When picking a clinic near you, just be sure to check out the reviews online before scheduling. (By the way, Mrs. Tancura says she'll answer any questions about skin maintenance for every ethnicity.)

FEELING THE DERM

I highly recommend seeing a dermatologist for some of your skin's special needs, but how do you go about finding a good one? Reviews, referrals, and ultimately your own intuition will help you decide. We trans and cis women have that intuition; we inherently know when something doesn't feel right. You, too, can pinpoint lots of moments when something didn't feel right. I've run the gamut with doctors. Up until recently, nobody knew what trans even was, so I had to educate many of my doctors. Hopefully in your situation, it'll be easier. Find someone you trust or who comes highly recommended, hope that your insurance covers them, and make an appointment. You should go at least once a year, if only for a mole and skin cancer checkup, but more often if you have problems that require medical intervention. A dermatologist can usually also refer you to a good plastic surgeon, if that's the route you decide to go.

TIME IS ON YOUR SIDE

As long as you take care of your skin on a daily basis, staying committed to a regimen that best meets your unique needs, I promise you it will pay off in the form of glowing, beautiful, and age-defying skin. It's worth the investment of time, energy, and money to keep your skin as your most gorgeous asset.

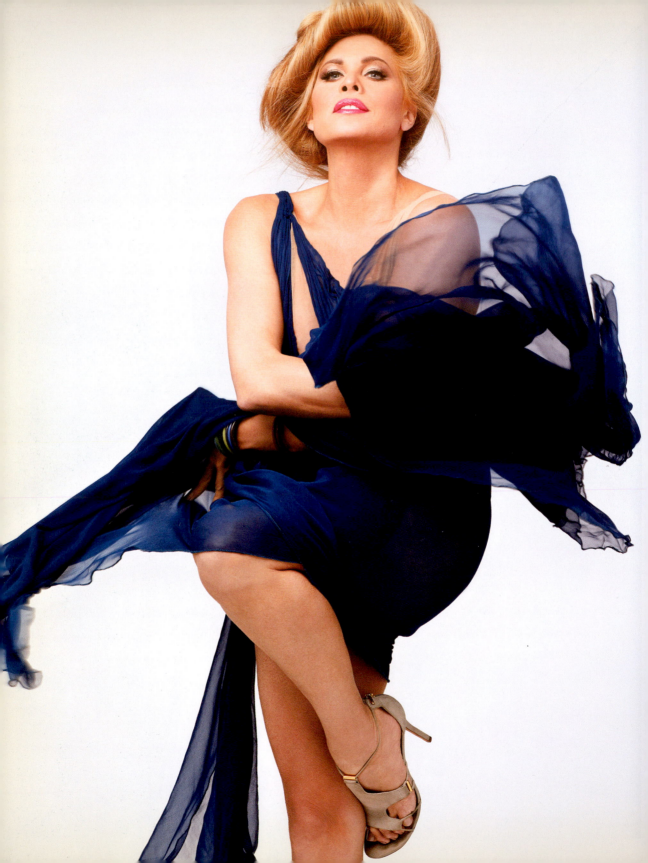

Part Two:

Giving Them the Highlights

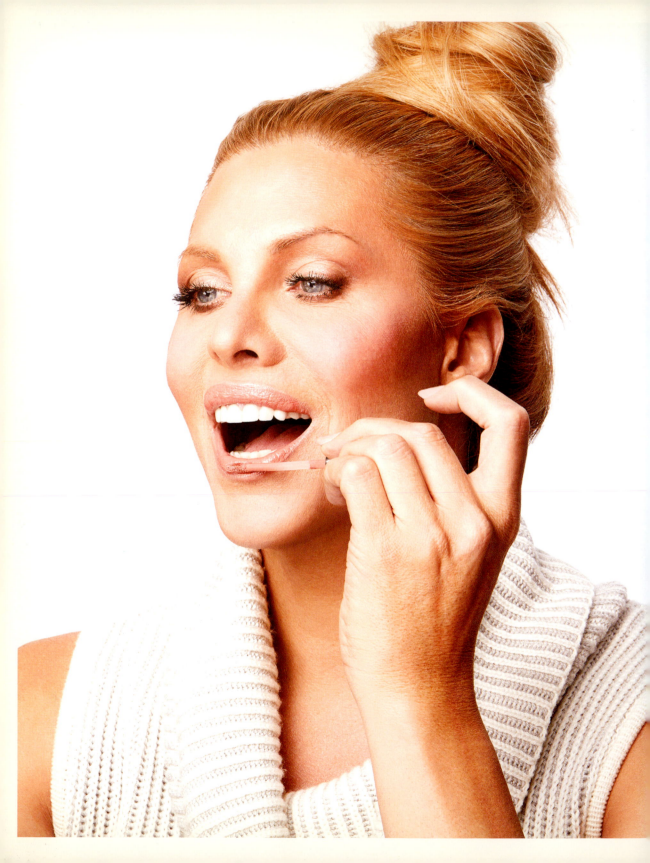

CHAPTER FIVE:
MAKING UP WITH
YOURSELF

"I BELIEVE THAT ALL WOMEN ARE PRETTY WITH- OUT MAKEUP— AND CAN BE PRETTY POWER- FUL WITH THE RIGHT MAKEUP."

—Bobbi Brown

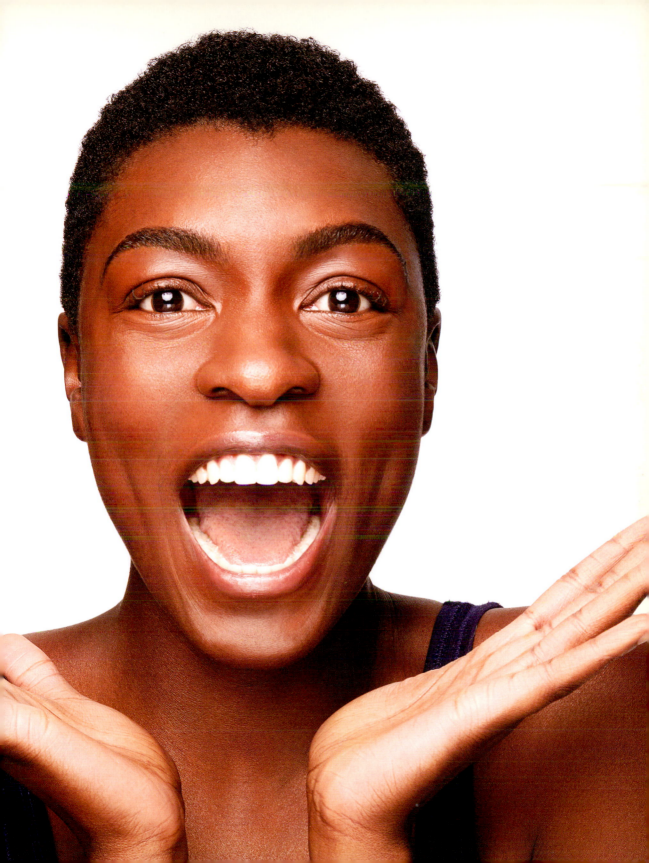

You may be wondering why it took all the way to chapter five to discuss makeup. That's because I truly believe you have to be 100 percent authentic from the inside out—so that your makeup becomes a reflection of the inner you versus turning you into an entirely different human being. It's all about letting your true colors come out to play with empowering makeup choices.

Makeup is what helped me to really see myself as authentically female. Of course, like any young girl, it was a total disaster when I first started playing with makeup, but I felt good experimenting and that's the most important thing. You learn as you go, right? I never stop learning from magazines, online tutorials, my "sisters," and professionals. It's good to let your beauty regimen keep evolving.

BRUSHES WITH GREATNESS

One of the most crucial elements of making up your own face is to use the correct kind of brushes each step of the way. There are four main groups: foundation, contouring, highlighting, and brow/lash. Foundational brushes have subcategories like concealer, blending/buffing, and applying.

Flat, rounded-off brushes are for applying foundation. Concealer brushes are smaller, flat, and rounded-off for greater precision. Blending and buffing techniques require a thicker kabuki brush. This is the classic brush we tend to think of with regards to makeup. It has a short stick with long, soft bristles that are light as feathers on your skin. They're wonderful for a sweeping, subtle application of powder, and the best kind to use for blush. They can also be used as highlighting brushes. For your brows and lashes you want to be extremely precise, so aim for a small, angled brush to fill in your brows and a brow comb that can also be used for eyelashes.

With contouring brushes, there's a whole lot to navigate and learn—but don't be intimidated, because I have a handy dandy cheat sheet on the subject for you:

- Small, tapered brush to contour around the eyes.
- Big, tapered brush to contour the cheeks and forehead.
- A specific nose-contouring brush.
- Crown brush to contour the forehead.
- Sponges to apply liquid foundation.

Watch a couple makeup tutorials and see how each one of these brushes is used. Check the Resources section (page 187) for links to some very helpful and informative ones. For highlighting brushes there are several different kinds, but most of them are pretty much the same. However, there are some smaller ones that can be used specifically to highlight the cupid's bow above the upper lip. There are also lip brushes, which are long and thin for more detailed work on a much smaller area of your face. It's great to have one or two lip brushes that can be used for blending when you contour your lips (more on that on page 83).

A lot of lip palettes come with brushes already, but if you're buying single sticks, lip brushes won't be hard to find—likely in the same section of the store. Trust me,

they're worth the investment when it comes to blending and shading those pretty little peckers.

There's one last step that is absolutely essential to the functionality of a brush: Care and upkeep. Above all, don't forget to keep your brushes fresh and clean to avoid the buildup of nasty bacteria. No one wants to use an old brush with caked-on foundation, blush, or lipstick. Rinse smaller brushes under hot water before each use, and the bigger brushes once a week with a cleaning spray. Leave them hanging upside down to dry overnight so they're ready to go the next day. Pretty simple, huh? Now that you're an expert at brushes of all kinds, we'll talk about the best way to put all these special tools to work—but first we need to prep.

PRIMED AND PLUMPED

Start by bringing your face out into the strongest, best possible light. To smooth out lines and bring your best face forward to share with the world, you're going to need a small collection of primers, concealers, fillers, and highlighters. Why do you need a primer, if you're already using a good foundation? Primer does for your face the same thing painting primer does for a wall: it covers up discolorations and creates a more solid and even base for your foundation to stay smooth (not shiny) all day long. Use it on your eyelids, too, before applying eye shadow.

Photo Finish from Smashbox or Burberry Primer are great primers that attract just the right amount of light to your face, illuminating it and empowering you to glow, but more economical brands, like e.l.f., makes very effective ones, too. If you have a lot of redness, Physicians Formula has a green tinted primer that will work harder to eliminate red patches.

because it gives me a bit more control and precision. You can use a small sponge to spread liquid concealer more evenly, if that feels best to you.

A FLAWLESS FOUNDATION

When looking for a foundation, don't be afraid to ask questions; go to a Sephora (or any makeup outlet) and ask for them to test your skin. Find something that matches,

Match your skin tone as closely as possible and be careful not to go too light.

Need to hide a little bit more? Concealers are made to provide additional coverage for areas of discoloration, so use these for under your eyes and on tiny blemishes for spot coverage. Match your skin tone as closely as possible and be careful not to go too light, because daylight will not be forgiving to that mismatch.

Looking for a respite from too many nooks and crannies? Plumpers and fillers are great for erasing deeper lines, bags under eyes, and crevices that you'd rather not be putting out there for general consumption.

As a general rule, I like to apply all of my primers and concealers with a brush,

and then get one shade lighter and one shade darker for highlight and lowlight purposes; these will help you to accentuate the positive.

The big question many of us ask is: Liquid or powder? I think it has more to do with the quality and consistency of your skin. If you have a lot to cover up and smooth out, a liquid will give you more coverage. If your skin is not as dependent on concealing flaws, a powder will do the job. Age is another factor; for older women with more "life lines," liquid foundation may come off as a bit too pasty—especially if you wear a lot of loose powder over it. Powder lightly if that's the case, so you don't run the

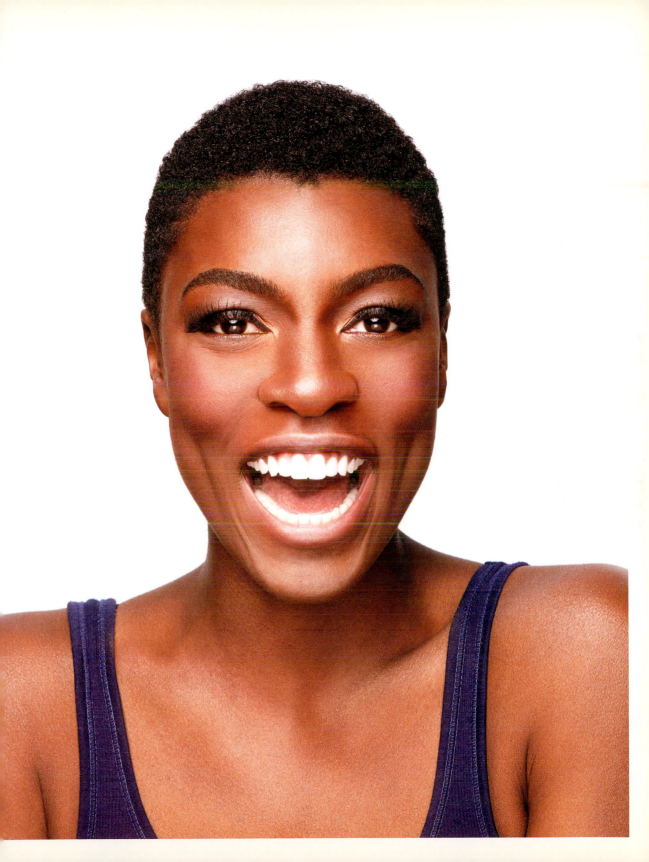

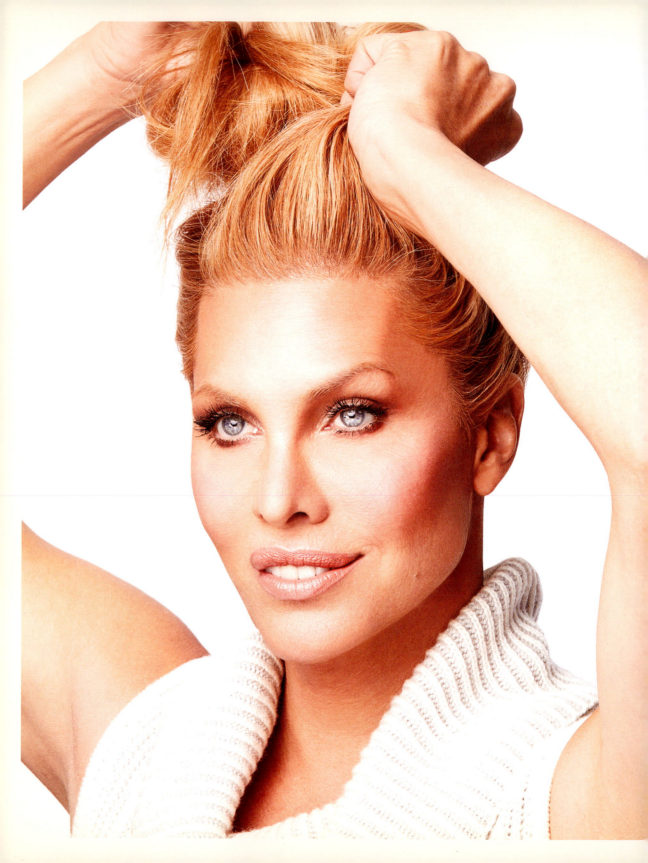

risk of making your face appear as though it is made of clay. For the silver foxes I recommend a nice, soft mineral powder to let your story shine through.

I use a Make Up For Ever Face & Body foundation, which is a more opaque foundation for daytime wear. At night, I'm not afraid to use a pan stick, (also from Make Up For Ever) and combine the two because you can get complete coverage and still have a "less-is-more" effect. It's a convenient way to do a "fast fix"—especially if you don't have much time between work and play.

To apply liquid foundation, use a kabuki or larger brush (or sponge), and dab only a dime-sized portion of the foundation on it at a time. Start with your forehead, and work your way down your nose, then spread out from there toward your hairline, ears, and neck. I set my foundation with loose powder; a light HD powder from Make Up For Ever for daytime, and for night I like to use slightly tinted Ben Nye luxury powder that comes in a multitude of shades so you can mix and match to get your perfect shade. After I powder, I use a powder puff to put a little extra powder under my eyes to catch specs of eye shadow that may have happened while doing my eyes. After you're done applying, you can easily brush it off with no awful shadow stains under your eye. (You can go over it with a light dusting of powder foundation to help it set even better—and then save some powder for going over your blush once you're done applying it later.)

Powder foundation is applied exactly the same way, only it's a bit faster because powder allows you to cover more ground at one time. With powder, be sure not to go too light in shade, or you'll look like one of those powdery doughnuts (which are delicious, just not on your face!).

CONTOURING 101

Everyone's always talking about contouring on social media, singing its praises and searching for different styles and techniques to create a seemingly flawless face. It can be challenging for beginners, but once you get the hang of it, it'll become second nature. Contouring uses the blending of different matte shades (nonglittery) and shadows to give your face and lips more definition and volume. The goal is to create a 3-D look with foundations and shadows that will leave your face glowing. It builds on the natural planes and proportions of your face and gives you a fresh, smooth, selfie-ready look.

Let's get your supply-list straightened out first. You'll need:

- Pan stick and liquid foundation
- Bronzer that is approximately one to two shades darker than your skin
- A sponge for liquid foundation and a flat or angled brush for powder
- A concealer or highlighter that is two shades lighter than your skin

There are different techniques for contouring different face shapes. Everyone's different, right? So it makes sense to have several

- The first step is super simple: just apply foundation to your face like normal, making sure to fully cover it with even, solid color.
- Next, add bronzer on your nose, over your cheekbones, under your hairline, and across your jawline. Be gentle and frugal with how much bronzer you apply—if you use too much you'll end up achieving more of a clown look than a natural one.

NEVER STOP BLENDING

When working toward your flawless finish line, the most important thing you can do is keep on blending. Starting in the middle of your face and working your way out into your hairline is the best way to avoid makeup lines—and nothing screams "amateur" louder than a premature finish line. It's easier to achieve a smoother, more complete finish with powder and a kabuki brush, but you can do the same with liquid foundation (as well as your blush and bronzers). The key is to create a soft, well-balanced, and completely finished look that leaves your face looking as naturally lovely as possible. We should never be able to tell where your makeup starts and finishes. We shouldn't be able to tell what's makeup and what's the real you.

different methods of applying makeup. I'm going to give you a basic primer (pun intended) on how to begin contouring, and when you're ready to get elaborate and take it to the next level, enter a quick search online and you'll find an entire treasure trove of contouring maps for each face shape. Until then, build your confidence with these basic guidelines:

- Dust some bronzer down your neck to create a smooth, blended gradient from your face to your clavicle.
- Add a light layer of highlighter or concealer on your chin, under your brow bone, under your eyes, over your nose, and between your eyebrows.
- Blend, blend, blend! Using either a sponge or brush, complete the contouring

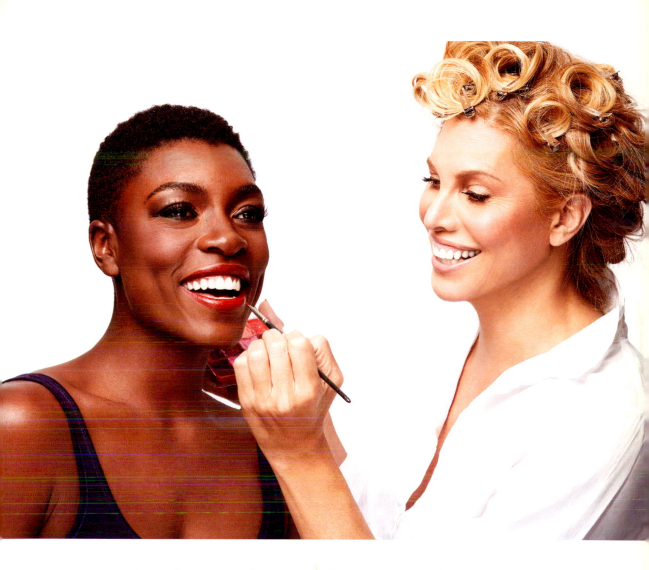

process with smooth transitions between each shade. Add eyeliner, mascara, and blush and you're all set!

• Finish the look with a light powder to seal the deal.

For a more dramatic look, contour in more areas of the face, like under your cheeks with a darker shade, or by your temples. (Caution: Don't add more or darker contour to just one area.) Most important, your goal is to accent your cheekbones and jawline. Show off those curves in your face, and I guarantee you'll see a big, exciting difference.

You can also contour your lips, if you're a lipstick-wearer looking for new ways to make your mouth pop and look fuller.

You'll need concealer, a lip liner, lip highlighter, and two shades of lipstick—one darker and one a shade lighter. Your lip liner should be a subtle shade or so darker than the lipstick—go for the same tone and color-scheme when choosing a lip liner and lipstick combos.

Apply concealer around your lips and blend it to the rest of your face. Then, outline your lips with your liner. Color in the outer edges of your lips with the darker lipstick, leaving the middle of your lips blank. Fill in the middle of your lips with the lighter shade and blend the two together until it's a seamless transition between both colors. Your lips will look positively plump and kissable.

It's easy to take your look to the next level with just a few tricks of the trade for contouring. You'll be surprised at how effortlessly gorgeous you can look when you master the art of contouring and use it to bring out your amazing, one-of-a-kind beauty.

MAKE YOURSELF BLUSH

Blush, gorgeous blush! While its main job is to add a natural color and glow to your cheeks, it can also add a little more

dimension to the contoured face. Color, consistency, and application are the big challenges for a lot of us, but here's how I think it can be simplified: When choosing your best blush color, my method is to hold it up against my skin in as natural light as possible. True complimentary colors will enhance the tone of your skin in a positive way. You can also apply it to the inside of your arm (near your wrist) to see how well it blends with your fairest skin tone.

For lighter skin tones, choose a soft pink or coral shade of blush; anything darker will come off as too orange or brassy. Medium skin tones do well with corals, deeper pinks, and plum shades. Darker tones can have fun with brighter shades of pink, coral, burgundy, or even purple—and if you add a splash of shimmer to it, your face will literally glow!

With blush, a little dab will do it; apply it with your brush in circular motions, starting just under your cheekbones and moving out toward your ears. For a more polished look, you can blend along your cheekbone with an angled brush.

Tip: The broader the brush, the less likely you're going to have sharp makeup lines; that's why kabuki brushes rock. Blend all of your borders with a kabuki brush, using a small amount of blush powder in a lighter tone.

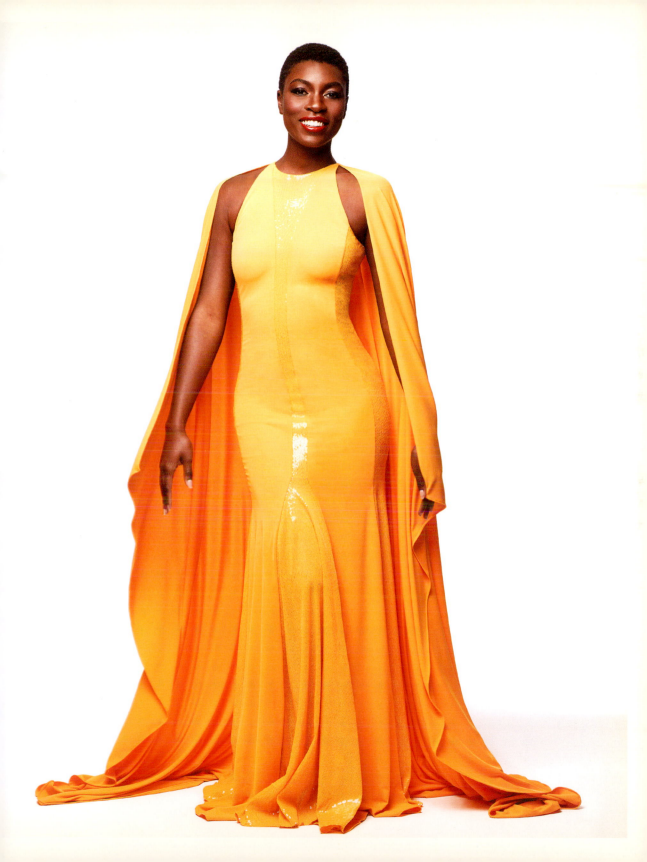

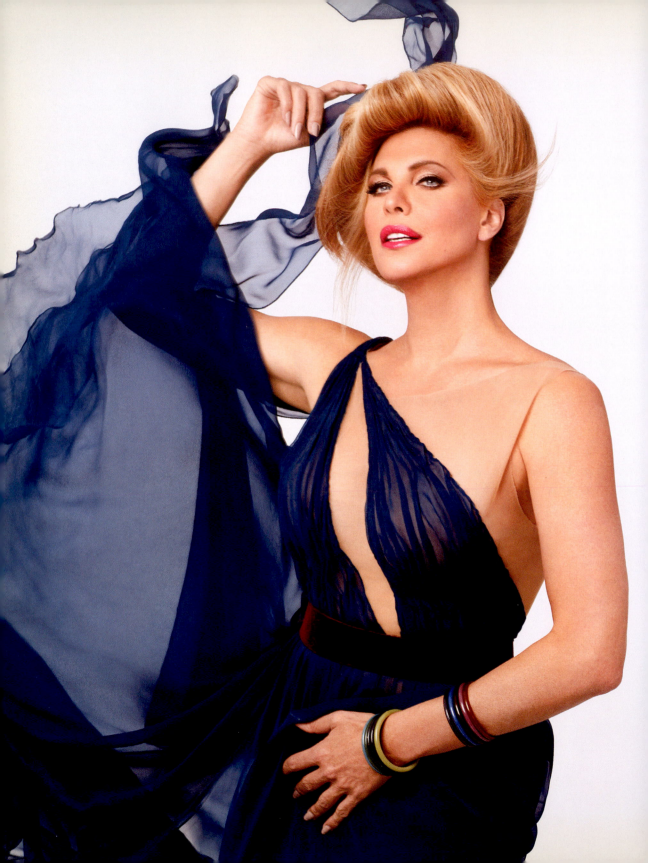

FINISHING TOUCHES

To finish off your best ever face, you can go outside the box to add a little bit more glamour. Glitter, shimmer, and a touch more bronzer are other ways to put your best face forward—and you don't need much of any to make let your inner light shine! Shimmers and highlighters usually come in soft, white, glittery shades—dip your brush into them, shake the brush off over the counter (or back into the container). You want to look like the glorious sun reached down and kissed you with just one tiny ray, not its full force. Apply shimmer to places where the actual sun would hit you—not your entire gorgeous face. That means midforehead, bridge and tip of your nose, tops of your cheekbones, and maybe a small dab on your chin. That's all you need to look like you are a true sun goddess.

MY "TOP 10" MAKEUP KIT

I use the same kit at home as I do when I travel. It has all the most important items. Just remember, your own kit doesn't have to be vast or super expensive:

1. Foundation
2. Loose powder (like Make Up For Ever's for day and Ben Nye luxury powder for night)
3. Eyebrow pencil
4. Six brushes (powder brush, contour brush, eyebrow brush, plus small, medium, and large eye shadow brushes)
5. Eye shadow selection (varies depending on season)
6. Liquid eyeliner
7. Lashes and glue
8. Blush and contour powder
9. Lip pencil selection
10. Lipstick

What are your most important beauty "rules"?

SCOTT BARNES:
"Always use body bling (my makeup product that's also a sun-kissed body lotion). It hides a multitude of sins and gives you that amazing glow all over. Why stop at your face, when you can do your whole body?"

JENNIFER RADE:
"Rules I never break: Don't line your lips in a color that doesn't blend with your lipstick. Blending is critical. And your eyebrows should not look they were drawn with a marker."

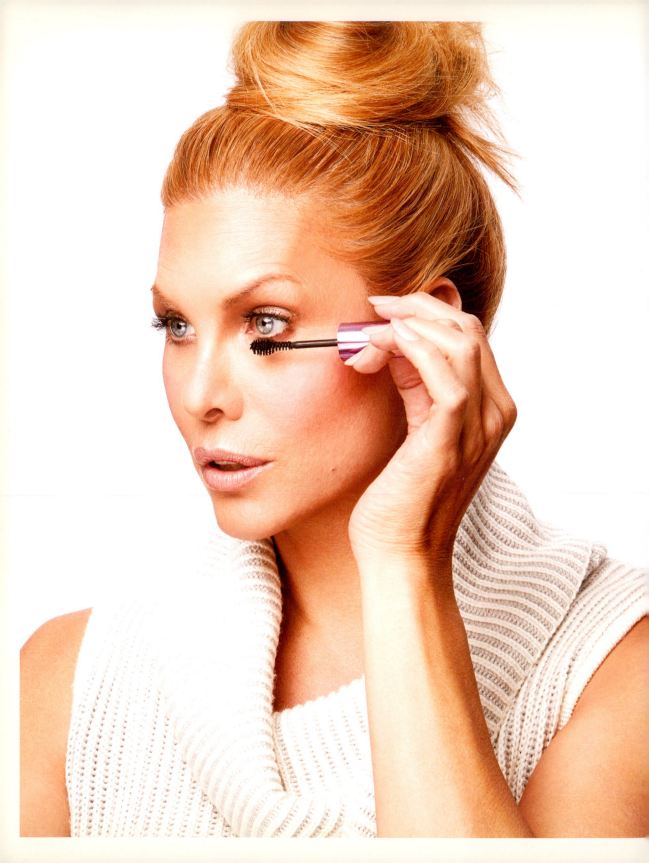

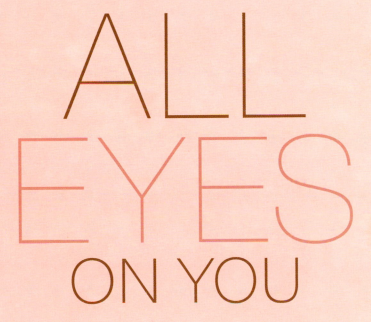

CHAPTER SIX:

ALL EYES ON YOU

"THE BEAUTY OF A WOMAN MUST BE SEEN FROM IN HER EYES, BECAUSE THAT IS THE

DOORWAY TO HER HEART, THE PLACE WHERE LOVE RESIDES."

—Audrey Hepburn

Eyes are the most expressive part of your face, and probably the most poetic, too. Imagine all the art that has been inspired by them—songs, paintings, photographs, and literature. They're really pretty magical, and the best part is that we all get to have that little bit of magic whenever we look in the mirror, or at each other.

So, how do we showcase them? Everyone's eyes are unique: different colors, shapes, and sizes. That's part of what makes them so special. We have to treat them with the utmost care and attention, because that's what they deserve—to shine as brightly as our souls. First, let's start by identifying your own one-of-a-kind eye type.

EYE OF THE BEHOLDER

Different eye shapes call for different applications. What shape are your eyes? Take a close look in the mirror and let's break it down. Generally, there are six types of eye shape: 1) monolid, 2) upturned, 3) hooded, 4) almond, 5) round, and 6) downturned. There are also close-set eyes and wide-set eyes. Don't worry, there aren't any tricks here—each type is exactly what it sounds like. Here's how to make each and every one of them pop while accentuating their natural shapes:

MONOLID: These lids are flat and creaseless, with a less-defined brow bone. The softer features of monolid eyes lend themselves to a variety of different looks. As far as the basics are concerned, you'll want to really define the upper lid with darker shadow and eyeliner, moving to lighter, shimmering shades as you go up toward the brow bone, to add more definition.

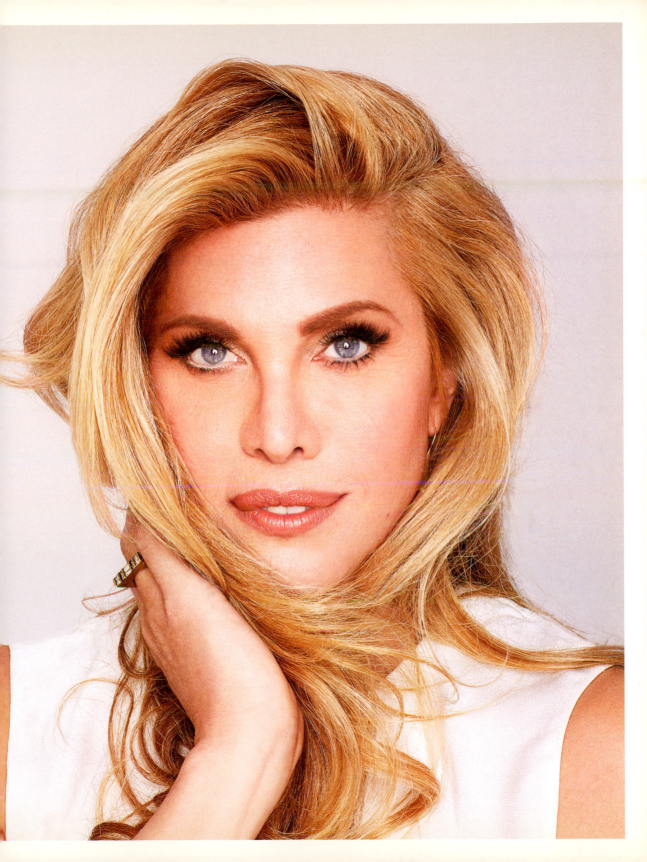

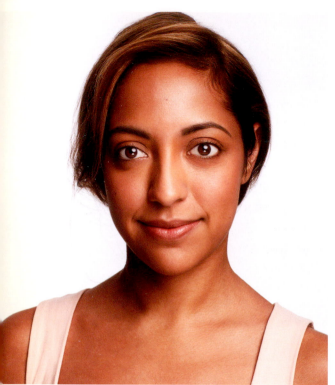

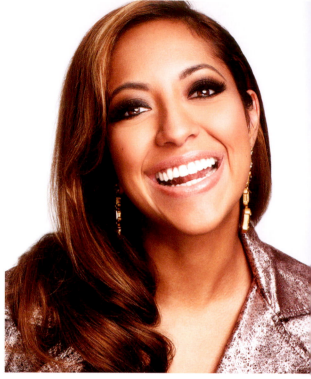

UPTURNED: These almond-shaped eyes lend themselves to more glamorous designs, with a sexy upturn at their outer corners. They work well with a gradient shadow on the upper lid, starting lighter at the inner crease and fading into a darker shade as the shadow travels to the outer half of your lid. This draws attention to the natural, feminine curve of your lids.

HOODED: With hooded lids, which have a little bit of extra skin over the crease and make your eyes appear smaller, you'll want to do everything in your power to brighten them up and give them a more dynamic

appearance. Darker shadows tend to work better for bringing out the shape of hooded eyes without highlighting their heavy lids.

ALMOND: Arguably the most versatile of eye shapes, the trick with almonds is to add depth. User darker shadows and line both your upper and lower lids to create a complete, polished look that makes your eyes pop.

ROUND: If you have round eyes, you'll want to put the most detail on your upper lid (to the brow bone) and leave your bottom lid more neutral or nude so as to avoid boxing your eyes in with a closed-off look. To make your eyes to look more full and spherical, definitely avoid liner on the bottom lid.

DOWNTURNED: These eyes run the risk of seeming droopy on the outer corners if not properly made-up, so your goal is to lift, lift, lift. You can do this by focusing most of your details on the top lid, just like you would with round eyes. Thicken your lashes, darken your shadow and liner, and leave your bottom lid light and neutral.

There we go! Easy enough, right? Now that we've covered the basic everyday looks, let's talk about how to make your eyes really sparkle.

THAT BRIGHT-EYED LOOK

Let's build from the beginning. Before we talk daytime or nighttime, we should start with some basic tricks on how to brighten your eyes and conceal that sleepy, "I-just-woke-up" look that we all have a tendency to develop throughout certain phases of our lives:

• Start with a good concealer or primer; apply it to your lid and undereye areas. Make sure not to go too light in shade, because that will give you the Tammy Faye Bakker (aka raccoon eye) look. It should be light enough to brighten your eyes, but not so much that the rest of your face looks like you spent too much time in the tanning booth.

• Apply your liner as evenly as possible; pull down on each lid to avoid broken lines from creasing.

• Just above your liner, apply a thin layer of some fun, light, and shimmery color (maybe an iridescent nude).

• Highlight your brow bone.

• Use a gentle and subtle nude on the rest of your lid.

• Apply a white (or nude) liner on your lower lash line for a wide-eyed look, or black or brown for a more sultry look.

• Highlight the inner crease of your eyes with the same iridescent nude as your lower lid.

• Put a dash of sparkly white, gold, or clear glitter next to the outer corners of your eyes.

    After those steps, add some mascara and you're all set! Awake, alert, and ready for the day—or, at least, that's what everyone will think (just kidding).

For a more casual daytime career look, here are some additional steps that make your eyes appear subtle, yet sublime:

• Go super light and subtle on everything. Remember, it's the office, not a club!

The goal is to be as natural as possible. This is especially true for you lovely older ladies:

- Add a little brown or bronze on the outer edge of your lower lid and fade into lighter shades as you work your way up to your brow bone.

- Define your brows with a little penciling and filling-in. Use a brow template (downloadable or sometimes included with brow makeup) if you need to create more due to a thinner brow.

This regimen will frame and enhance the natural beauty of your eyes, and look totally effortless by the time you're done. But what about when you're done with work for the night or for the weekend? There are endless gorgeous and elegant styles for nighttime eyes, but a timeless classic is, of course, the smoky eye. If you're ready to master this sexy look:

- Start with a nude base as a primer over your entire lid.

- Add a light layer with a "smoky" color (dark gray, dark brown, or black) over the entire lid.

- Darken the smoky color toward the outer edge of your lid.

- Highlight the inner crease of your eyes with a silver or light nude.

- After your lid is done, you can put a liquid liner above your lashes for a more

dramatic look; to tone that down for a softer, yet still dramatic look, put a brown eye shadow over the liquid liner; it will temper the dramatic but add depth.

- Highlight your brow bone.

- Add liner on both lash lines

- Apply two to three coats of mascara on the top and bottom lashes. If you are blessed with a nice, full set of your own lashes, simply apply some mascara from lid to tip on your top lashes, and only do the tips of you lower for a more natural (and less spiderlike) look.

All right, smoky eye all-star. Go hit the party scene, and take lots of selfies! And guess what? You now have three different, yet complimentary makeup tricks for all hours of the day. For special occasions, you can simply build off these three styles—add glitter or fun colors. Experiment and have fun. Check out Pinterest and YouTube for some really fantastic tutorials (including my own—at www.candiscayne.com).

CELEBRITY EYE CANDY

What kind of eyes does your favorite celebrity have? Which celebrities share *your* eye type? Identifying your eye type with a celebrity can be a pretty useful trick when it

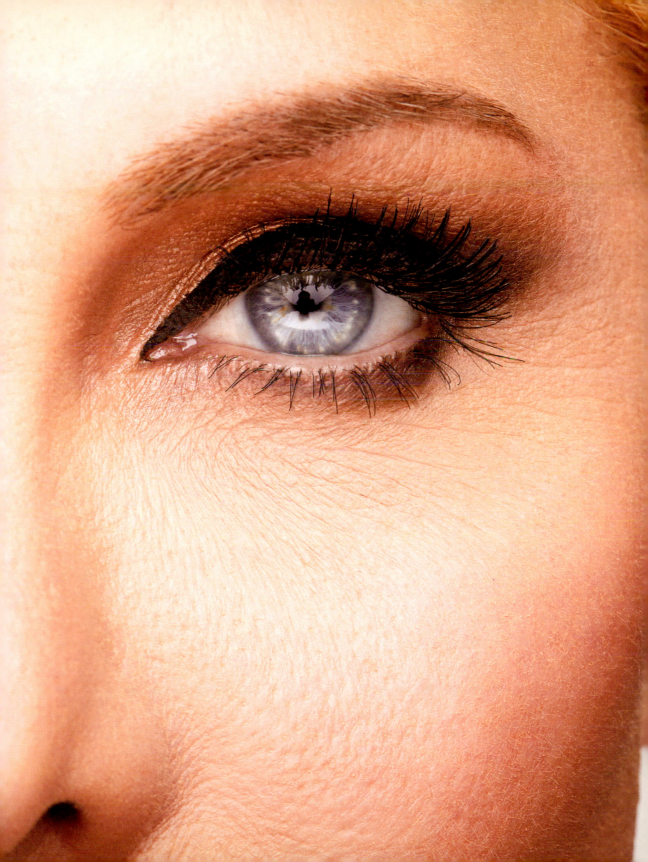

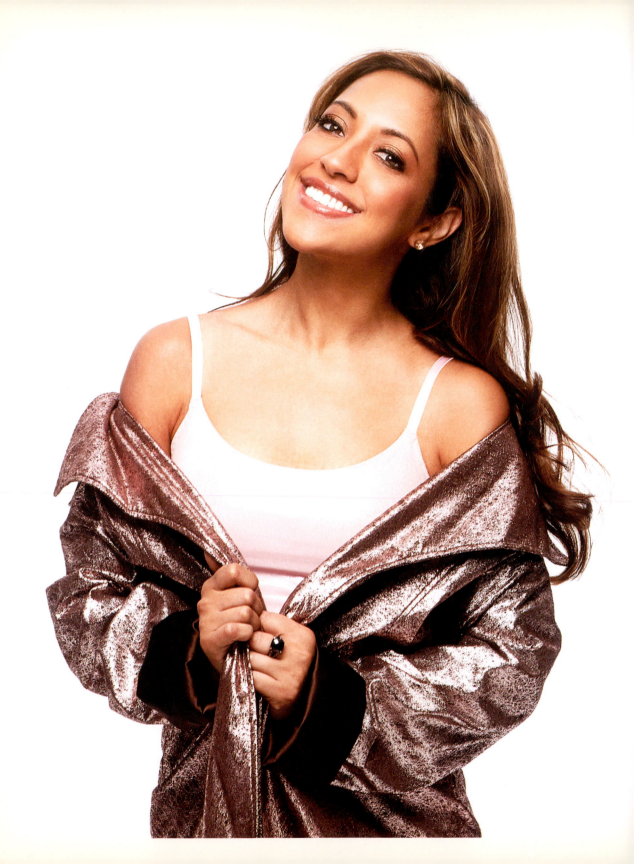

comes to makeup ideas. Celebs have super-expensive, high-end stylists and makeup artists who are especially devoted to making their clients look red-carpet-ready on any given day. Check out their photos—their Instagrams, Twitters, and image search results on Google. I guarantee you'll find some exciting and glamorous looks to experiment with that will leave you looking ready for your close-up, too! Here's the celeb "A-List" for all eye types, to get you started.

MONOLID: Sandra Oh, Yuna Kim, Lucy Liu, and Jamie Chung

UPTURNED: Angelina Jolie, Sarah Hyland, Mila Kunis, and Rihanna

HOODED: Beyoncé Knowles, Sofía Vergara, Taylor Swift, and Blake Lively

ALMOND: Jennifer Garner, Olivia Wilde, Megan Fox, and Penélope Cruz

ROUND: Kerry Washington, Emmy Rossum, Katy Perry, and Zooey Deschanel

DOWNTURNED: Anne Hathaway, Tiffany Hines, Katie Holmes, and Eliza Dushku

No excuses! Now you've got a celebrity cheat sheet. Use it to your advantage and turn up the glamour.

FRAMING THEM UP

There are ways to match glasses to your face shape and look totally classy and glam while wearing them.

OVAL FACE: Go totally wild. I'm not kidding! Oval faces are super flexible when it comes to choosing bold and distinct glasses. Whether it's artsy, chunky frames or some thick cat eyes, your face will thank you for some fun and unique accessories. The sky is pretty much the limit (lucky girl!).

ROUND FACE: The key is to accentuate your shape with strong, defined glasses that sit off your cheeks (i.e., with nose pads) and are wide—to add dimension to your

AN EXTRA LIFT

I like to embellish with the individual clumps of false lashes instead of applying a single set of false ones. It only takes me a few minutes to do all of them, but I have lots of experience now. For those of us with less-than-stellar lashes, there are products that lengthen with microfiber and give thin lashes volume and drama. They're great, but if you want less fuss, try and just curl your lashes—it brightens your eyes with no product at all. You can even use a small amount of Vaseline on the ends to keep them curled and separated.

For accentuating your eyes with eyeliner, remember that less is always more. Unless you have a specifically dramatic look in mind, lots of liner around your eye can make them look smaller, so be careful. I usually do a liquid liner on my top lid and a little shadow underneath my bottom lashes. Also, if you want to tone down a dramatic upper liquid line, grab a thin brush and go over it with a dark shadow; it softens the edges and makes the line less severe.

I'm a fan of a thicker eyebrow nicely manicured and arched. Superthin, round eyebrows were last seen in 1936, so please be gentle with your tweezer.

cheekbones—rather than tall, which tends to make your face seem shorter.

HEART FACE: Because your lower face and chin are narrower than your forehead, your goal should be to keep the details of your glasses on the bottom, and aim for a broader, wider shape on top. Your frames can be darker in color, but try to blend or complement your hair and eye color.

SQUARE FACE: Avoid boxy or square glasses and instead go for a rounder, thinner, and subtler shape. Since your face has already got some delicious angles, you'll want your glasses to be softer, both in frame and color.

As far as colors are concerned, you'll want your glasses to match the majority of your closet. With that in mind, go shopping at your local eyewear store and find your perfect match!

For you colored contact lens wearers, choose an eye color that complements your skin and really makes your eyes pop in a gorgeous way. Generally speaking, the darker your skin, the more vibrant the lens color can be. Violet eyes like Elizabeth Taylor's can be worn by women with lighter skin. Express yourself through your eyes; let them speak their truth through a wonderful shade of you.

Accentuate your look with a dramatic pair of sunglasses for the ultimate daytime look; hey, when you're cool, the sun is always shining, right?

COMMUNICATING WITH THE EYES

Did you know that there are real, scientific ways to read someone's eyes? I'm not talking about metaphysical methods. You can tell a lot about a person—especially how they feel toward you—just by the movement of their eyes. For example, if you're talking to your crush and you notice their eyes dilating, that's a good sign that they really like you. Light comes into our eyes through our pupils, so the wider the pupils get—well, "the better to see you with, my dear!" However, if you're talking to someone and their eyes dart around or seem unable to focus, that's probably an indicator of anxiety or distracted thoughts, and that's *not* such a good sign because it means either the person is focused on their own issues, or just plain not into you.

As far as your eyes are concerned, it's impossible to tell whether or not your own pupils have actually dilated appropriately (should you be talking to someone you like), but you can try a couple of other eye-language tricks to make your intentions known. If you want to send your crush some signals, try maintaining eye contact for a few seconds, look away, and then look back. That indicates a cute shyness mixed with bravery. Eye contact can be scary; let them know you mean business without seeming overly aggressive or confrontational. Too much steady, unbroken eye contact may creep them out or send the wrong signal. Be careful, but most important, have fun, take risks, and bat those lashes like you mean it, girl!

IT'S ALL IN YOUR EYES

Ultimately, your eyes tell your story. That's why it's important to frame them as authentically as possible, so they tell the truth about you and enable others to see you for who you really are. Whether it's for a date, a job interview, or just plain, everyday living, it's important to be as honest and open as possible so you can shine your light not only on everyone you meet in life, but also on those who are fortunate enough to be sharing it with you already. You are beautiful and don't forget it—your eyes certainly won't. And now, with all the tools and helpful tips provided in this chapter, you'll have everything it takes to make them shine just a little bit brighter (especially for that special someone). Feeling more confident yet? Just wait until you put it all together, look in the mirror, and be inspired to take a few dozen selfies. That thought won't seem funny once you start seeing yourself with new eyes. Who says you need a celebrity stylist to look like a star? With the right makeup, and in some cases, glasses and contacts, you'll look like you just left the set of a photoshoot. So, get going! Be your own celebrity stylist. You have everything you need to help your face glow like the sun in its own, special, way.

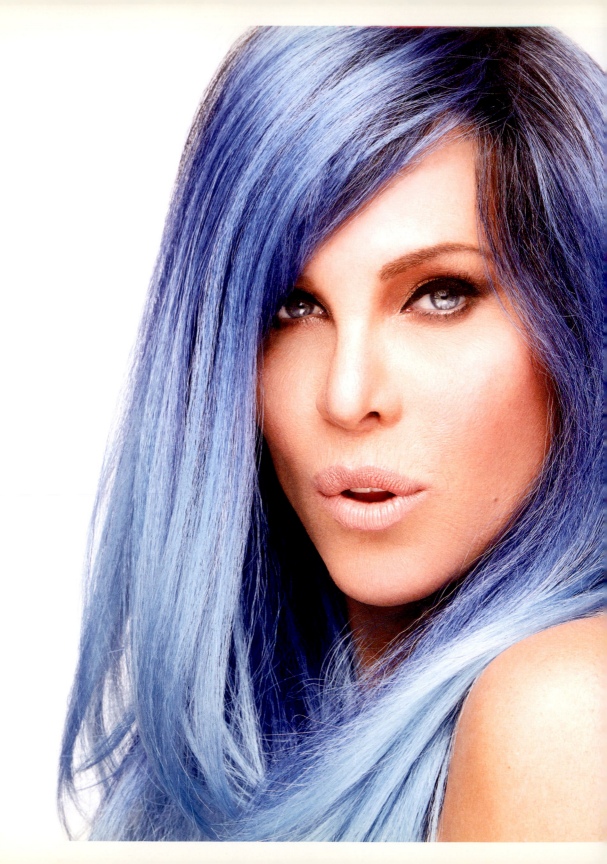

CHAPTER SEVEN:

BLOWING KISSES

"THEY PRESSED UPON HIS BRAIN AS UPON HIS LIPS AS THOUGH THEY WERE THE VEHICLE OF A VAGUE SPEECH; AND BETWEEN

THEM HE FELT
AN UNKNOWN
AND TIMID
PRESSURE,
DARKER THAN
THE SWOON OF
SIN, SOFTER
THAN SOUND
OR ODOUR."

—James Joyce, *A Portrait of the Artist as a Young Man*

ere's a little secret: lips can be the most voluptuous part of the human body. They are full of blood, nerves, and energy centers that enable your body to feel all kinds of wonder, especially in the middle of an amazingly tender kiss. Yet, too often, they're an afterthought: The last thing you do before going out is slap on some lipstick, purse your lips together, and dash out the door. They're worthy of so much more attention, so let's all do what Lauren Bacall said when instructing Humphrey Bogart how to whistle in the classic film *To Have and Have Not*: "Put your lips together, and blow"—then wet your whistle with the very best products, colors, and treatments you can muster, to create a smile that can literally transform your life.

LIP CARE 101

Let's start at the very beginning of good self-care for your precious pout. Did you know you can exfoliate your lips, too? Buy a lip exfoliator (they're inexpensive—or you can even use brown sugar mixed with honey or olive oil), and use it about once a week. You'll love how soft and sexy it makes your lips feel—and it's great for removing any chapped or dead skin on or around your lips.

Next, nourish and protect your lips. I know I've said this before, but here we go again: Water, water, water! Staying hydrated does the absolute most good for your lips, and helps keep them from getting chapped often, especially in the colder seasons. Eat healthy fruit and vegetables for a steady influx of the right vitamins and minerals into your system, which will strengthen your lips and make their natural color more vibrant. If you're eating right, you might be

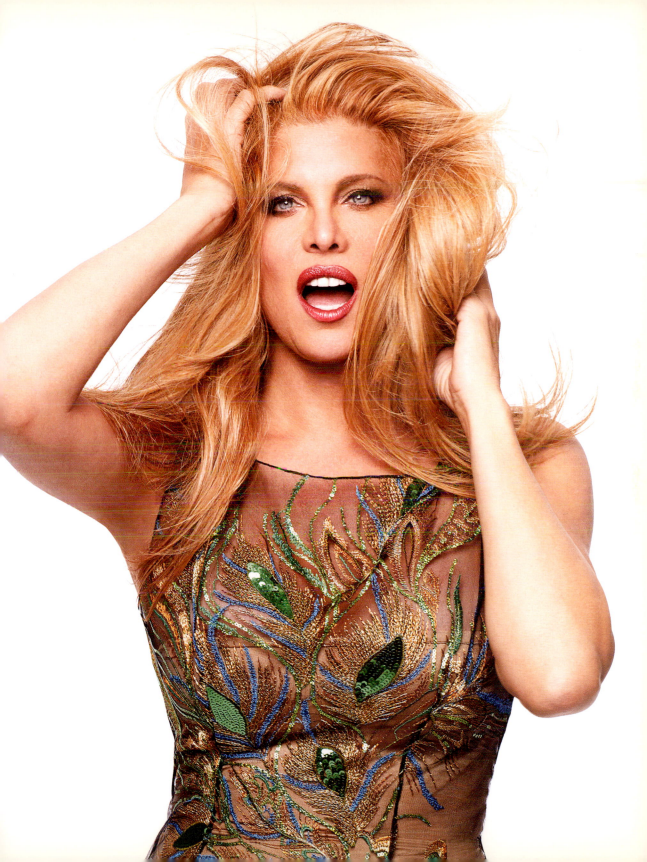

in the enviable position of being able to get away with only a dash of clear lip gloss—at least for your daytime look.

Choose the appropriate balm for your lips based on your skin needs. Beeswax, paraffin, olive oil, jojoba, and aloe vera are the best ingredients to look for in a hydrating, softening lip balm. SPF should be a minimum of 15 to protect your precious lips from the harsh rays of the sun. You can use a Vitamin E–fortified balm, but don't depend on that alone to do the hard work of keeping your lips soft and supple.

THE ULTIMATE LIP WORK-POUT

Surprisingly, you can change the shape and fullness of your lips by doing some sim-ple exercises. Since they are totally free, it's worth a shot before you seek out more extreme methods. Here's how to give your lips a "work-pout":

- Fold your lips into themselves to stretch the skin around your lips, and help to minimize wrinkles.
- Pucker your lips, hold for five to ten seconds, and then release with a huge smile. This will stretch the skin on your lips and help strengthen your lip muscles.
- Purse your lips together and lift them up toward your nose. Hold for five to ten seconds, then release and repeat.
- Using your (clean) fingers, stretch the sides of your mouth; apply some lip balm to the corners of your mouth before and after.
- Suck on an ice cube, or use a straw to exercise your mouth's muscles.

TO ENHANCE, OR NOT?

As I've said, I'm not opposed to the use of Botox or other plumpers when it comes to filling in lines or enhancing problem areas. However, when it comes to lips, I think it's best to try as many natural approaches as you can before turning to outside help. Botox can plump up your lips, but it can also weaken the muscles in your face—and that can result in the dreaded "Joker" face. Try using cosmetic plumpers, lip liners, and the like to make your lips appear fuller. If nothing else seems to work, then you can call the dermatologist for options.

How do you know when to stop plumping? I always think that making little enhancements are okay, but it's important to plump gingerly. You can achieve a fuller look without making yourself look obviously plumped.

In acting class, we also practice saying certain words and sounds, like "Oooooo," "Ohhhhhhh," and "Ahhhhh" and then begin annunciating words for clarity and simply to get our mouths engaged in the scene. You don't have to be onstage to do these exercises; you can practice the same ones, just to improve your presentation skills and be better understood.

LIP LANGUAGE

Your lips don't just help you get the right words out; sometimes, they speak volumes on their own:

SLIGHT SMILE: "You amuse me."

SEXY SIDE SMILE: "You intrigue me."

FULL-ON WIDE SMILE: "I really enjoy being around you."

LAUGHTER THROUGH SMILE: "You are so funny!"

TWISTED TO ONE SIDE: "I don't have a clue what you mean."

TIGHTENED LIPS: "I'm not sure about you."

FINGER TAPPING LIP: "I just might . . ."

POUT: "I'm not happy" (or, possibly, "I'm just playing").

SCRUNCH: "I can't make up my mind."

Make sure you're telling the right story with your lips, or you'll be sending mixed messages. It's amazing how often people mis-read intentions based on misunderstood lip language. Set the record straight—or keep your lips sealed.

THE DIRTY, SEXY LIP LIST

Okay, since I was featured on the show *Dirty, Sexy Money* (and kissed a Baldwin boy, just sayin'), I couldn't resist coming up with my own DSL list. What lip types do your favorite celebrities have? Which celebrities share *your* lip type? Line yours up to theirs to find lovely lip inspiration:

ANGELINA JOLIE: What else can I say? She has the best lips in the business, and uses them to create more good in the world. That's literally putting your money where your mouth is, am I right?

EVA MENDES: Exotic, voluptuous lips accentuated by a beauty mark.

SOPHIA LOREN: Italian perfection.

AUDREY HEPBURN: A timeless, classic beauty with soft, lovely lips.

LAUREN BACALL: A thin upper lip to add mystery, over a full lower pout. No wonder Bogart couldn't resist her.

MARILYN MONROE: Red lips were never the same after her. The beauty mark made them stand out even more.

SCARLETT JOHANSSON: Her lips are almost round, like a cherry. Any color looks

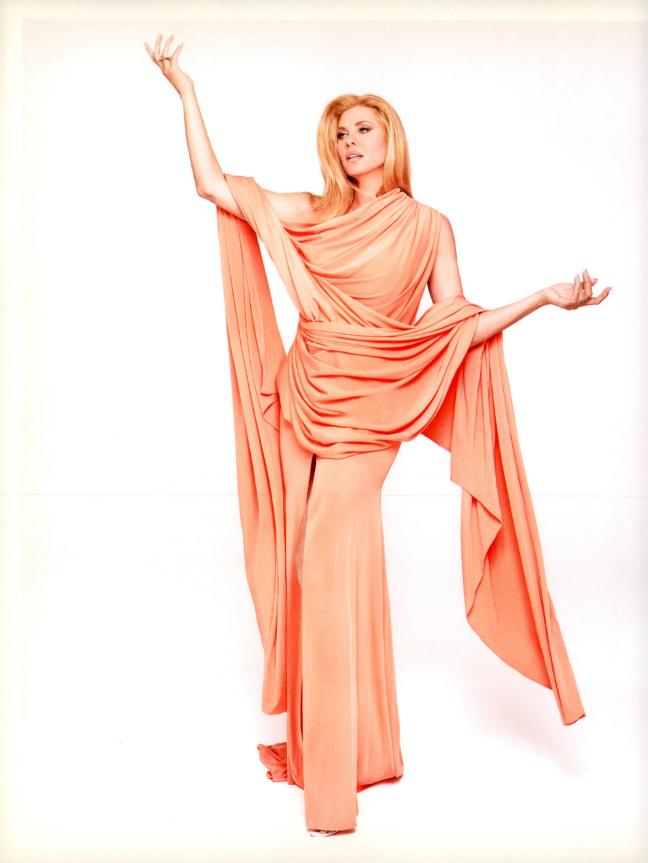

great on her, and her smile shows it.

LUCY LIU: Her top and bottom lips are also in perfect proportion, giving her a fierce smile.

DITA VON TEESE: Classic, burlesque-style beauty—with lips that evoke memories of Hollywood's Golden Age.

KERRY WASHINGTON: Lips that could put an end to any Scandal—or start a whole new one.

LUPITA NYONG'O: Gorgeous, full lips and a skin tone that reflects her inner light; this is why adventurous lip colors totally work on her.

OPRAH WINFREY: Warm, caring, inviting lips that let you know that she is listening to your every word.

IMAN: Perfect proportions all over that gorgeous face. She uses vibrant, unusual colors to highlight her lips.

LINE AND SHINE

Lots of women ask me how I feel about liners versus a natural look. During the day, I mostly like to wear a clear or slightly pigmented gloss, but other times I line my lips and fill them in with the liner almost like a lipstick. I leave a space in the center to add lipstick or gloss for a gradation.

Liner can definitely be used to your advantage. If you have thin lips, use liner to fill in and give your lips fullness and depth.

If you already have fuller lips, you can use it lightly to accentuate. Start at the corners and move inward toward the center; if the center is very light, apply slightly more lip liner to that area to give more fullness. For drama, fill in entire lip area; for subtlety, apply it in light, feathery strokes. Try to create curves or a sense of movement wherever you can.

For your overall lip look, let's look at colors. While traditional shades that match or complement your hair color and skin tone (not to mention your outfit) work best for the majority of us, it's okay to experiment with some bright, fun colors, too. Generally speaking, the younger you are, the more you can experiment safely with neons, bright purples, and even orange lip colors. For older women (unless you're an Internet sensation like Baddie Winkle!), stay away from the loud shades in favor of lighter, more natural-looking, choices that give us a hint that you may be up to something. When you're experienced, you don't need to advertise it, right? Here's a quick color guide for the pout-perplexed:

REDS: Darker reds with blue tones work well on darker or olive skin; darker-skinned African Americans, you lucky girls look great in any color. Bright orange red looks great on fairer skin, although Stila makes a matte red called "Beso" that weirdly works on almost everyone!

BERRIES: These can be worn by women of any skin tone or hair color; here, it's more about lip shape. Those with thinner, lighter lips can use berry tones to make them stand out more.

CORALS: Redheads with light skin, or dark-skinned women with full lips, can pull off corals brilliantly.

PINKS: Pretty much anyone can wear pink lipsticks; it's just a matter of how deep or bright the pink. Softer pinks look better on blonde, blue-eyed ladies; brown- and black-skinned women can look fantastic in bright pinks.

METALLICS/BRONZES/COPPERS: These glowing shades really pop on redheads, or women with warmer, darker skin tones.

DARK BLUE OR BLACK: Unless you're a lighter-skinned woman going for a goth look, or in your twenties, these are much more dramatic on darker-skinned ladies. I've seen some redheads pull it off successfully, but blondes just look like Harley Quinn and they're too overpowering for lighter brunettes.

THE JOY OF LIP ART

What about trying a really fun look, like lip art? There are tons of great Pinterest boards with ideas ranging from rainbow and pure gold lips to fruit, ice cream, candy, and even floral looks. You can be as trendy as you like, but try to use these looks for outings where they will be best received: cons, beauty shows, and club nights. These looks can be quite distracting at the office, so keep your more classic looks going there. For added dimension, match your lip art to your nails and outfit, and then dab some sparkly white glitter-based eye makeup to the outer corner of your eyes. If you're not a good artist with a steady hand, make a design template to follow or have a friend do the artistic work for you. Be sure to capture some good photos of it, too, because you'll want to remember how to recreate your look in the future.

I have seen a few women who have gotten tattoos on the inside of their lips,

MATTE OR GLOSS?

Matte is great for a serious, or more dramatic, look and it's really hot right now—but a touch of gloss can add some glamour for a night out. A simple layer of gloss alone (or with a neutral color) can give you a soft, pretty daytime look.

or tongue piercings. If that is what helps you to more fully express your true self, it's okay; just don't do anything that extreme if you aren't willing to live with it for a very long time. Lip piercings can be well done or over done; choose these wisely. The best ones are small studs or rings that can be removed or swapped out on a regular basis, to keep your look fresh and more adaptable to your outfits. Of course, you can remove a piercing and let it close up if you decide you don't want it anymore, but a tattoo is harder to remove, especially in the mouth or facial area.

PEARLY WHITES

I live in Los Angeles, where nearly everyone has beautifully white teeth. I'm sure that some go to their dentist to have it professionally done for hundreds of dollars, but you know what? With all of the great self-whitening products in drug stores today, it's relatively inexpensive and easy to accomplish pearly white teeth at home. Crest makes a number of effective whitening products, as do many other manufacturers, and you can buy everything from a simple toothpaste that whitens over time to dental office-quality whitening trays. If you're not sure what to use, ask your den-

tist for suggestions. It all depends on how much staining you're starting with in the first place. If you've got a lot from coffee and smoking, you'll need professional assistance; if you already have some whiteness and just want to enhance or protect it, then toothpaste will do it for you.

Gums also require attention, since gingivitis can lead to bad breath. Probiotics and baking soda with peroxide toothpaste can really help you build stronger, healthier gums, keeping your breath fresher while limiting decay over time for a beautiful smile to grow old with.

Calcium helps keep your teeth strong as well. Just take the daily recommended amount, and don't overdo it because it can build up in your system and cause other worries.

What about veneers? Honey, if you need them and can afford them, they are worth their weight in gold—mainly because they will make you feel more confident, and more likely to flash your winning smile. Implants can do that, too, so they are always worth it if you've lost any teeth.

MOVING IN FOR THE KISS

Nothing—and I mean it—is a bigger turnoff when it comes to kissing than bad breath.

You're all set to kiss that person you've found so exciting, and when you get to the point of contact, you catch a whiff of garlic. Or is it onions? Or sardines? OMG, make it stop!

To keep your own breath fresh and inviting, start by brushing your teeth. Floss, and then rinse with a mint-based mouthwash (preferably with natural ingredients versus an alcohol base). Some dentists rec-

ics or probiotics made especially for mouth issues. Cutting back on carbs like pasta can also help eliminate bad breath, since foods like that turn to sugar in your body, and create a sugary aftertaste. If you're dining out, be sure to make use of that little garnish that good chefs put on your plate; chewing on a little sprig of parsley or mint is a great way to freshen your mouth while you're away from home.

GLAM ON THE GO

s it ever too late for braces? Not with the new InvisAlign technology available. You can have your teeth straightened, without anyone noticing. Just remember to practice speaking, because these invisible braces often cause a temporary lisp that will make you sound like Cindy Brady. It takes a few days to get used to them, but don't worry—your tongue will get the hang of it quickly.

Don't lick your lips too much, because it dries them out—and so does breathing in and out through your mouth instead of your nose.

ommend regular tongue scrubbing using your toothbrush; it's a good idea unless you have a sensitive mouth, in which case, use a baking soda or peroxide mix to gently scrub your tongue.

Breath mints and gum are good for in-between brushes and cleanings, but these are temporary fixes and more or less like applying a Band-Aid to a wound. If you have breath issues, you need more help than that—maybe even oral antibiot-

One more thing: replace your toothbrush every two months or so in order to limit bacterial growth.

Now here are my tips for giving (and receiving) the best kisses:

• Close your eyes. Enjoy the moment by closing off your visual senses for just a moment, to allow your lips to do all of the feeling (except for the occasional peek, because it's kind of sexy to look at).

- Pucker up—but not too much. You're not kissing grandma here.
- Don't slobber. Being nervous can lead to increased saliva production, and that can be a huge turnoff. Relax, breathe, and let your lips do the work. I once broke up with a guy because his spit was always dripping down my neck. Ewww.
- Don't limit yourself to kissing only on the lips. Let your lips do the "talking." If you're going to do a French kiss, use the tip more than your entire tongue.
- Be natural! Nobody likes to kiss somebody who is stiff. If you feel way too nervous, it may be a signal to wait; something might be off, and you want it to all be right, right?

Finally, and this probably goes without saying, don't kiss anyone who has even a small cold sore on their lips; that's how cold sores spread, and some can result in very nasty infections. You don't want the kind of "gift" that keeps on giving like that, right?

Kissing can be one of the most pleasurable experiences we can have as human beings, and that's why it's important to take good care of your lips. You never know when you're going to meet someone who makes you quiver—but if your lips are in the best possible shape and look inviting, the pleasure will be worth all the effort it took to make them that way. So, pucker up, buttercup. Kiss long, hard, and passionately—and your lips will love you forever.

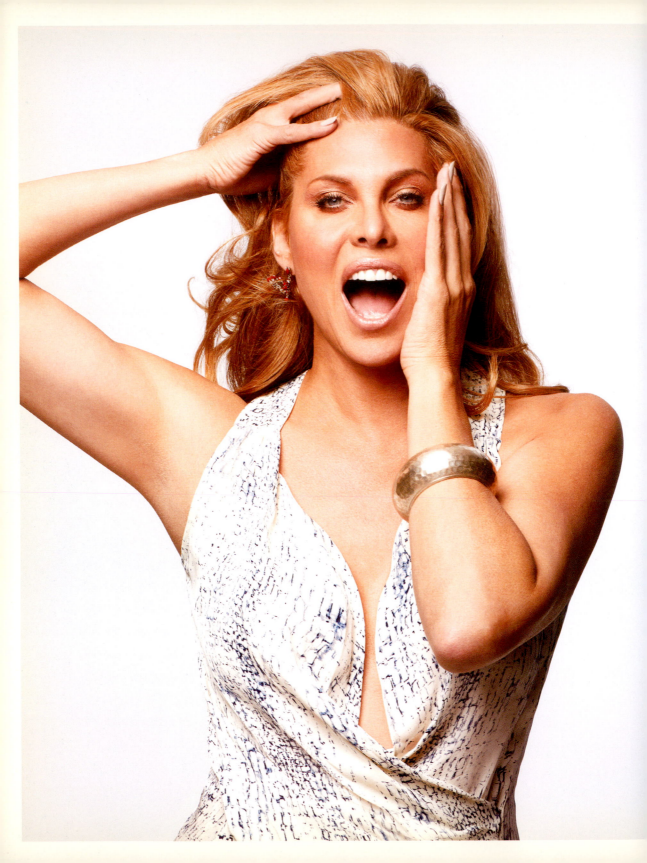

CHAPTER EIGHT:

NAILIN' IT

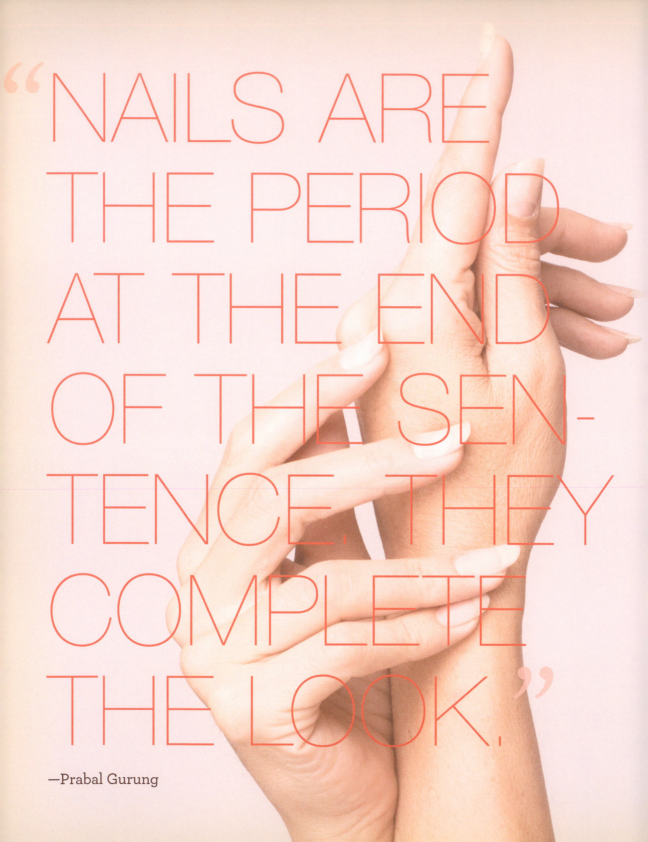

"NAILS ARE THE PERIOD AT THE END OF THE SEN- TENCE. THEY COMPLETE THE LOOK."

—Prabal Gurung

id you know that some of your greatest fashion potential is at the end of each of your fingertips? Whether they're your favorite indulgence or, sadly, your makeshift chew toys, nails are the beginning and end of every outfit—a bookend that both accentuates and completes your look. What's more, nail art is always individual to the unique fashion expression of its wearer.

Whether it's for a red-carpet event or for a night at your bestie's house, painting and decorating your nails is a very intimate and special art form—one that deserves to be studied, practiced, and perfected. Remember: Your nails are an extension of you, and just like every other part of yourself that you decorate, you want to be honest and truthful, so you can shine your brightest light from the top of your head to the tips of your toenails.

So many people overlook the visibility of their nails, but their style, color, and shape are of the utmost importance when it comes to really and truly putting your best "you" forward. So, let's get started!

FIND YOUR SHAPE

First things first: you need to correctly identify your own individual nail shape. This is the "natural" shape of your nails without any alterations. If your natural nail shape is not the one you want, don't stress— it's easy to switch up at home with clippers and an emery board, or, of course, at your favorite salon. There are five basic fingernail shapes for you to compare your own nails to and, if you'd like, to model your own dream nails after:

OVAL: Like its namesake, the oval nail is comparable to the round nail, but longer and slimmer. It is the ultimate delicate, flirty, and romantic shape, and would do well with very feminine shades (pinks and nudes) and embellishments.

SQUARE: Bold and strong, the square nail is exactly as it sounds. Women with this shape are often born leaders, and their nails would look best with colors that showcase their trendsetting nature (vibrant reds, blacks, and purples).

SQUARE OVAL, OR SQUOVAL: A hybrid between the square and oval shapes, the "squoval" is round and slender around the base and middle, with a contrasting straight-edge top. This shape is great for ambitious women who mean business and aren't afraid to show it. Think professional, solid colors (darker reds, blues, and browns).

ROUND: The all-around classic round nail is perfect for the born intellects. With the conservative round nail, your best bet for colors are more fall-inspired (browns, golds, and blues).

ALMOND, OR POINTED: For you divas and starlets, the almond or pointed nail is totally your type. These are trendy and brave shapes that not many can pull off; if you're one of the lucky few who

can, you better flaunt it with some unusual and wild colors (metallics, neons, or glittery)!

Now, just because these five nail types are "natural" doesn't mean that their shape and style can't be duplicated, even if your own shape is very different. Before you start snipping, though, remember that *all* nail types are beautiful and fun in their own way, and you should make sure that you try working with what you have first. There are plenty of wonderful tutorials on Pinterest and YouTube for how to trim and shape your own nails (or go to my website at www.candiscayne.com)—but, if you're feeling extravagant or just want to pamper your-self, the nail salon will do it for you.

THE LONG AND SHORT OF IT

After figuring out what nail shape you have (or *want* to have), the next big step is determining what length you want your nails to be. This is critical and should depend largely on your everyday lifestyle. If you're an active person, go for a short style, unless you want to be repairing split nails every time you get home from the gym. If you want pointy or square, make sure you can still function normally without straining

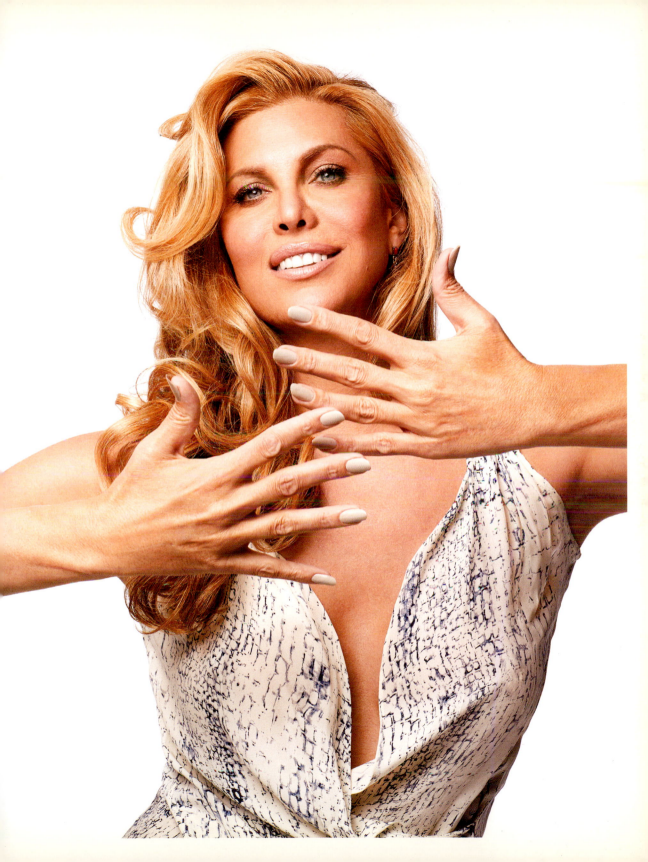

because of your nail length. For example, can you comfortably type on your keyboard or on your smartphone? If the answer is no, I'd suggest taking a little off the top. Unless you're a total long-nail or fake-nail pro, in which case, keep on keepin' on!

Glamour is always a plus—but you want to be practical, too, and there are plenty of ways to be practical *and* glamorous. I tend to go for a rounded medium-length nail. I'm active, so I keep my nails long, but not long

even down to your fingers and toenails. That's the key to everything, isn't it?

DEFINING YOUR DIVINE COLOR

We know what colors best match our nail shapes, but what about other deciding factors, like the seasons, holidays, or special events? Well, no matter what time of year

It is so important for you to know and love every part of your body as intimately as you can.

enough for them to get in the way. With a medium-length nail, you get the best of both worlds: they're long enough for you to easily experiment with colors, patterns, layers, and even adhesives—but they're not so long that they complicate your everyday routine. But, if you're really into the long, runway style, be sure you do your research on how to keep your nails happy and healthy, whether you grow them out yourself or apply fakes. For instance, from a nutritional standpoint, Vitamin E can help grow healthier hair and nails. Also, nail and cuticle oils help prevent brittle nails, and give an assist to nails that just don't seem to grow. Long, short, or medium-length, the most important advice I can give you is to take care of and love every part of yourself,

it is, I say be bold. Wear whatever color you want and make a statement. I wear all types of color, and I always do a pedi at the same time. It's always a wonderful feeling to have all your fingernails and toenails fancied up at the same time—even if it's wintertime and your feet are covered by socks during the day, it can make you feel special and glam just knowing your toes are secretly beautiful underneath all that fleece. You don't have to choose the same colors for your fingers and toes, either. Get creative and edgy. Who said you have to match? When it comes to fashion and art, there really are no rules. But there are some helpful tips that will aid you in starting up your own special palette for any event in any season:

FALL: Try burgundies, navys, and browns for a sophisticated look that will go perfectly with any sweater or knit pullover and will look gorgeous while holding your favorite hot coffee. The seasons are changing and so are you, so reinvent yourself with a delicious, dark, and velvety smooth shade.

WINTER: Go for blues, grays, and purples. Add sparkles for flair—and some metallics and glitter, too. Make it a "winter wonderland!" Mirror the snowy skies and twinkling stars with a little bit of bottled, sparkly magic. Darker colors + sparkles = your very own starry night to "wow" everyone with whenever you take off your mittens!

SPRING: The earth is awake again and flowers are in bloom, just like your fresh, new style. What colors do we want to see most in spring? Light, bright, flirty, and floral. Dark colors are out and pastels are in. Embrace your inner flower child and give your nails that lush, vibrant, freshly fallen petals vibe.

SUMMER: The pool is open, the sun is out, the sunscreen is on sale, and your nails are itching for a new look. Cherry red, lemon yellow, watermelon pink, tangerine orange—are you sensing a theme, here?

Your nails will look so juicy you'll want to take a bite out of them. Go vivid. Be an eye-catcher. Just in time for a summer romance, right?

HOLIDAYS: This is where it gets crazy. If you look for "holiday nail patterns" online, you'll get thousands of swatches and tutorials on how to complete the ultimate holiday look. Whether it's sparkles and gradients or stick-on reindeers and snowmen, you'll be more prepared than anyone for a holiday party.

SPECIAL OCCASIONS: This depends heavily on the event, but a good rule of thumb is to stick to nudes that can easily match any gown or outfit, and can be built upon with jewels, crystals, or even other paints. With a strong, neutral base, you can go a long way.

When you have the right palette, you can match any color in your wardrobe to a complimentary color on your nails. You'll always have that finished, complete look.

FINGER BLINGIN' GOOD

What if you want to take your nail art a step further? I remember in the 1990s when I worked for Patricia Field, I started gluing

Swarovski crystals on my feet one by one till they were covered. It looked so good that everyone wanted them—so much so that Pat asked if I would start a nail bar. You can be artsy and creative with your own nails, too. There are plenty of nail-adhesives such as rhinestones and decals that can take your look to the next level. In the spring, instead of just painting your nails pink like rose petals, you can actually place tiny roses (in the form of nail decals) on your nail. How cool is that? Not to mention you can put an *entire* other nail on as an adhesive, if you don't have time to mani/pedi yourself at home. The possibilities are truly endless. The more you experiment, the more fantastic your nails can look no matter what the season or occasion. You can buy really exciting decals and stick-on gems online. The alternative is, of course, to get fake nails or adhesives at your favorite nail salon. But if you're strapped for cash, there are plenty of cost-efficient accessories even at your local Target that will put you in the Instagram mood.

YOUR AT-HOME MANI/PEDI

For those of you teaching yourselves how to do a home manicure or pedicure, don't worry—it's a lot easier than it sounds. Sure, when you go to the salon you get the full, (potentially pricey!) treatment, complete with a massage and fancy oils, but just because you don't have an on-call masseuse with sugar scrub doesn't mean there aren't ways to pamper yourself at home. Getting to see your own hands and toes in a new light is a wonderful exercise in self-love and self-exploration. Get familiar with the way your skin cradles your nails, how smooth your heels are after you exfoliate them, or what parts of your hands get dry during the winter. It is so important for you to know and love every part of your body as intimately as you can. That'll make the process of giving yourself a relaxing home mani/pedi even more special. Ready to try it? Feet first!

- Make sure to remove all your current nail polish, if you're wearing any.
- Soak your feet in warm, soapy water with Epsom salts for five to six minutes. This softens your skin and makes it easier to scrub off calluses and push your cuticles back.
- Trim your nails to the shape you want them, then push back your cuticles and remove the excess skin.
- File and buff the edges of your freshly cut nails.
- Scrub and exfoliate your heels and behind your toes. Don't use the so-called "cheese grater" tool for this process, as it

can seriously hurt your skin. Instead, use a nice, natural pumice stone to smooth over your rough edges.

- Rinse your feet and apply lotion all over them, and up your calves.
- Dry your feet completely with a towel.
- Apply one even layer of base coat to your nails.
- Then, add the nail color. Apply two to three coats of color, depending on how vibrant you'd like the shade to be.
- Once the color has dried, put on one even layer of top coat, and voilà! Home pedicure achieved.

"So, Candis," you're saying, "that was easy enough. But what about manicures?" You're right—manicures are a little trickier, because not all of us are skilled with both hands. It can be done, though, as long as you're slow and steady. The steps are similar to home pedicures, but some are in a different order.

- Remove all your old polish.
- Trim, buff, and file your nails.
- Soak your hands in warm water with Epsom salts for three to four minutes— enough time for your skin to become softer, but not wrinkled.
- Push back your cuticles and remove the excess skin.
- Apply a healthy coat of lotion over both your hands.

- When the lotion dries, apply a base coat. Make sure there is no oily residue left on your nail, or the polish will not stick.
- Add the nail color in layers, just like your toes, depending on how vibrant you want the shade to be.
- Wait for the color to dry and then add a top coat.

You did it! Pretty easy, right? To keep it looking fresh and salon-quality, keep moisturizing your hands and feet every day and touch up your color when you need to. You've got some valuable information and skills now, girl. Before you know it you'll be giving all your friends in-home mani/pedis, and they're going to love you for it!

PAMPERING FROM THE PROS

If you do feel in need of a professional mani/pedi—which, let's face it, we all do sometimes—then there are a couple things to keep in mind before you hit up the salon. We all want a safe, clean, and friendly environment to relax in. Some of you may already have your go-to salons, but for those of you who are new to this type of pampering, there are a few things you'll want to do before you make any appointments.

First, check a salon's online reviews. See what kind of ratings they have locally, and what people have said about them. Take it all with a grain of salt, though, because not everything on the Internet is true. But pay attention to repetition: if the same pro or a con is consistently listed in multiple reviews, then that might be a good indicator of its truth. Once you weed through reviews and narrow down your list, you'll want to find out the health standards at each salon—do the technicians wear gloves, do they use single-use emery catch any and all red flags that way—plus, you'll get a good tutorial on how professional mani/pedis are done, and you can duplicate it at home!

Professionals can also come to the rescue during those times when your own nails just aren't working with you. You might decide to go for something like an acrylic or fake nails so that you can experiment with all the fun colors and styles that you aren't able to with your own natural nails. Lots of people do this, and it's very stylish. Have you ever tried acrylics?

GLAM ON THE GO

When you go to a salon, invest in a hand and foot massage in addition to getting your nails done. It feels so good, and will help stimulate the blood vessels in your hands and feet. Guess what? That will also help your nails grow.

Along with a healthy diet, supplements can also help your hair and nails to grow. NatureMade Hair, Skin, and Nails is a popular one that you can easily find at any grocery or drugstore.

boards, how do they disinfect each station? Usually it's pretty easy to tell how clean a salon is just by walking in. Really, the only thing you have to do is pay attention. If it's your first time at a salon, the best advice I can give is to be interested in what your nail tech is doing. Ask questions, make conversation, or just observe quietly. You'll If not, there are some general precautions that will help keep your nails underneath healthy and firm for all you fashionistas out there thinking about getting them.

• Keep your nails clean before each appointment at the salon. This, of course, is a no-brainer. You don't want to run the risk of trapping dirt or grease under those acrylics. There are some things that even the salons miss!

- Find a good salon and stick to it. Being a regular somewhere makes it easier to trust your nail tech and feel more at ease. Treat your nail tech like your personal stylist, because that's truly what they are.
- Be prepared to commit. Acrylics are not only expensive and require frequent upkeep, but they can also weaken your natural nails underneath, to the point where they break and have to be removed or filed down. It'll take some time for your natural nails to build up strength again, so be sure that when you commit to acrylics, you're in for the long haul.

Acrylic nails have incredible and enchanting designs and colors that just aren't always possible with natural nails. Though they're a big commitment, they're a perfect fit for some people.

THE A-LIST FOR YOUR "A" GAME

There are good nail polishes and then there are *great* nail polishes, and all of them are easy to find at your local drugstore or beauty shop. The top three polishes I'd recommend are Butter London, Essie, and OPI. One of the things they all have in common is their proud "3-free" or "7-free" status—which essentially means their polish is free of the three biggest and baddest chemicals typically used in other nail polishes, and some are free of an extra five more.

- Butter London 7-free polish contains vitamins that nourish and strengthen your nail as you apply it. It's bright, vibrant, and completely safe. In fact, it's *good* for you.
- Essie 3-free polish is incredibly stylish, trendy, and long-lasting. There are hundreds of colors to choose from this line, and they have a rotating seasonal collection that will always keep you ahead of the game.
- OPI 3-free polish is in high demand due to its huge catalogue of colors, both limited edition and year-round. It's smooth, safe, and beautiful. What more could you ask for?

If those three don't do it for you, other non-toxic polishes include Deborah Lippmann, American Apparel, Julep, and wet n wild.

So, are you ready to open your own nail salon yet? You've got what you need to be a rock star at nail art. Pick some fun colors, research some eclectic patterns, and glam yourself up—from your fingers to your toes. You've nailed it.

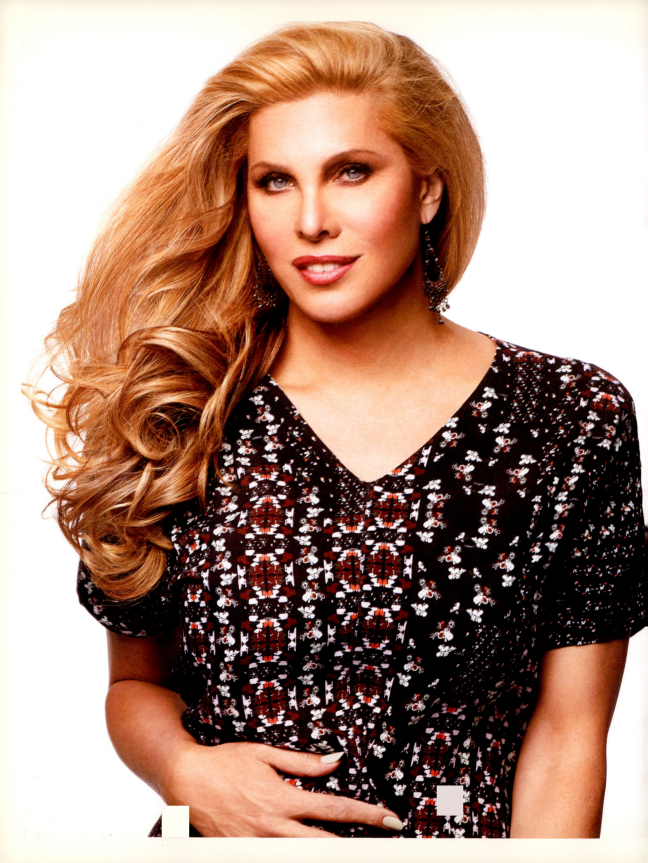

CHAPTER NINE:
YOUR CROWNING GLORY

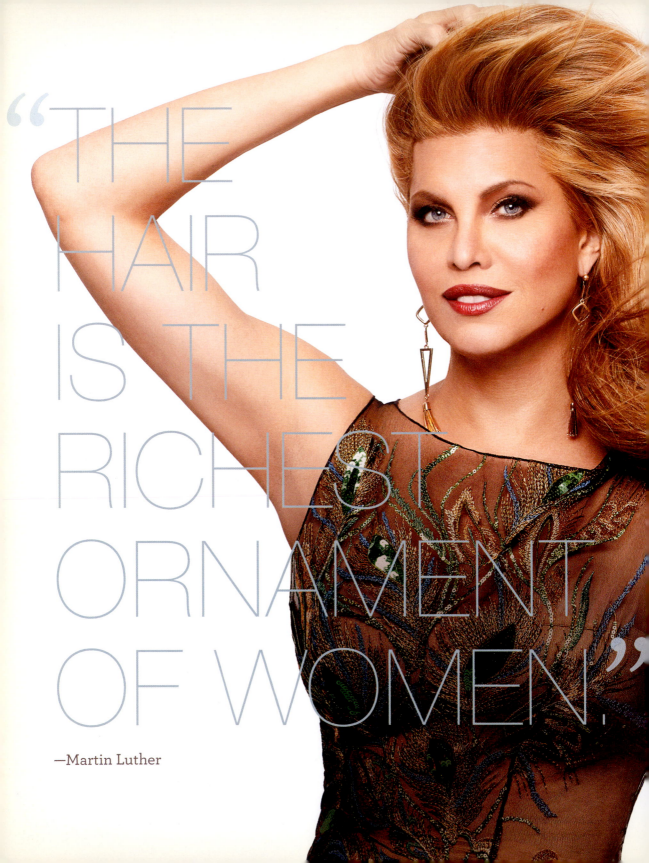

"THE HAIR IS THE RICHEST ORNAMENT OF WOMEN."

—Martin Luther

air is one of my favorite topics, and I have a lot of experience with it. Actually, I'm kind of known for mine. A lot of it is genetics; I got my thick hair from my dad. He's seventy-five and still has a full, thick head of hair. The cut and color come from me and my stylist (and best friend) Danna Davis.

I learned hair styling early on, pretty much the way we all do, by watching and practicing. Throughout the years, I've tried all sorts of colors and cuts, and ultimately I found the look that works best for me.

There are so many exciting ways to use your hair as a form of expression: Texturing, razor cuts, undercuts, asymmetrical cuts, and more colors than there are in the rainbow are available today, giving you the opportunity to use your hair as expressive art—a self-portrait that you carry around on your own head.

For you, gorgeous ones, the first thing to do is to figure out is whether you're a short-, medium-, or long-hair person. Some women can wear any length, but most of us have one length that really favors us by framing our faces elegantly.

Remember, your hair is one of the first things that people see when they look at you—so you'll want a style that looks good and, more significantly, makes you feel beautiful, powerful, and confident all the time!

CARING FOR HAIR

The single most important thing you can do in order to have gorgeous hair is to learn how to take good care of it. In a lot of ways, that is simpler than you think:

CLEAN: If you have very short hair, you can wash it daily—everyone else needs to take a chill pill and do it every other day. This will give your hair a chance to regenerate its own natural oils, which in turn will keep it vibrant, healthy, and growing. Use sulfate-free shampoos that contain more natural ingredients (like olive oil). Change your products frequently so your hair doesn't get too used to one pH level.

CONDITION: Keeping your hair conditioned will help stop breakage, hair loss, and split ends. Conditioner makes your hair softer and shinier, too. You can do a deep conditioning treatment on the off-day from shampooing, or use a leave-in

TOOLS OF THE TRADE

It's really important to have the right tools for the job. My own must-haves include a three-quarter-inch curling iron; hair oil for texture and shine; Bumble and Bumble Surf Spray or some kind of salt spray for a windswept and natural "beachy" look; and dry shampoo to lift roots for a fresh look between washing.

I also like a boar bristle brush, which will smooth the cuticle of your hair, so it will appear shinier and smoother. Metal

Wear your hair however you like to express your inner goddess—but some styles are more flattering than others.

conditioner over the weekend if you don't have any big plans. By the way, contrary to popular belief, conditioning is for your scalp, too.

PROTECT: Color your hair with hair-friendly products (not just anything from the drugstore); twist it into a bun or let it air dry, at least every now and then; use protective products, especially before using a hot curling or straightening iron. Protect your hair from the sun's harmful rays with a baseball cap (for more active exercise like hiking or biking) or a straw hat with your beach outfit.

barrel brushes are better for curl and volume. You should have at least one round and one flat brush—and don't be afraid to skip the brushes sometimes, if your hands can get the job done just as well. The more natural, the better—and that applies to hair more than any other part of your beauty regimen.

For detangling, a comb that has multiple rows was literally made for the job, so invest in one.

A scalp massager can be very comforting, but it can also help stimulate follicles to keep your hair growing.

Get a spray bottle and keep it filled

with some hydration mineral mist, or just some water and a small amount of conditioner, to spritz on your hair throughout the day and keep it looking and feeling fresh.

Finally, invest in a drawer full of clips, bobby pins, scrunchies, hair bands, and other accessories that can help you create new looks. Collect looks you find and create a Pinterest board—then experiment with your "drawer of tricks." The more you play, the more looks you'll find that you can create for yourself. Take selfies of the ones you like the most.

FRAMING YOUR FACE

Your face is a work of art, sweetie, so frame it with the right style based on your face shape. Here are some ideas for the five basic face shapes:

OVAL: You are the most blessed being of the hair universe, and can wear any style, any length, at any time. Feel free to experiment, and change your look often.

ROUND: Shorter hair will make you look too round (though I think this look is especially beautiful on Asian women). Stick with chin-length or longer, and frame your lovely face with some textured bangs, a few layers, and maybe a side sweep. Use a root plumper to gain some height.

SQUARE: Your longer face will be best complemented by longer hair, so go long and strong! To soften your face, go with a blunt cut and use a round brush to curl your hair inward, toward your chin. Use a side part and tuck one side behind your ear to add an air of intrigue to your look.

HEART: You can wear longer styles, as long as you layer or texture your hair—but really, you will rock the shorter, razor-cut, and undercut styles. Also, you are the absolute Queen of the Pixie.

DIAMOND: You are a medium-hair mama, so roll with it. Keep it midlength, curved under with a round brush, and add some dimension with an asymmetrical cut.

BANG IT OUT

When it comes to bangs, those of you with square-shaped faces need to proceed most carefully; shorter bangs will make your face look more extreme, so keep them long and wispy—and ideally swept to one side. The same is true for diamond shapes. Ovals and hearts can beautifully sport any length of bangs; however, they do look their best when they are layered or angled. Round faces are best framed by longer, side-swept bangs; straight, blunt-cut bangs will make you look like a toddler.

YOUR HAIR PERSONALITY

Of course, you can wear your hair however you most like to express your inner goddess—but there are some styles that are simply more flattering than others. The funny thing that I always hear about hair is that everyone wishes what they don't have: If yours is straight, you'd rather have curly; if it's red, you'd rather it was blonde, etc. But the truth is, not all of us look (or feel) our best with short hair—and that's because of your face shape as much as it is about your personality. Are you more of a pixie in your daily life? Then go with a short cut. Short hair is usually quick and easy, but you don't have the option of just putting it up when you don't feel like washing or styling it. When you get up in the morning, can't get a shower, and are already late taking the kids to school, short hair can be as scary-looking as bedhead!

Are you more free-spirited, flowing, and hippie-like? Then you know you're a long-haired girl. Long hair only looks good if it is healthy and frizz-free, so make a commitment to taking really good care of it.

Are you a traditionalist who's obsessed with classic looks? Go midlength, or choose a smart bob. Your hair should not only complement your face, it should also go perfectly with your personality for the most unified look achievable. Whatever you choose, here are some basic guidelines:

Sexy short hair tips:
- Timeless looks include a wedge cut, razor cut, and the bob (avoid "helmet head" at all costs).
- Use a round brush to make your hair seem fuller.
- Apply Be Curly from Aveda to accentuate natural curl.
- Condition your hair every day to keep it healthy and untangled.
- Have fun with color and shape (highlight with a splash of vibrant color).
- Keep your length in good proportion to your face length and shape.
- Maintain your cut every four weeks (including shaving neck).

Marvelous midlength tips:
- The lob (or midlength bob) is the most flattering look for you.
- Add a lift by back-combing at the crown; pull sides back with bobby pins, or tuck one side behind an ear.

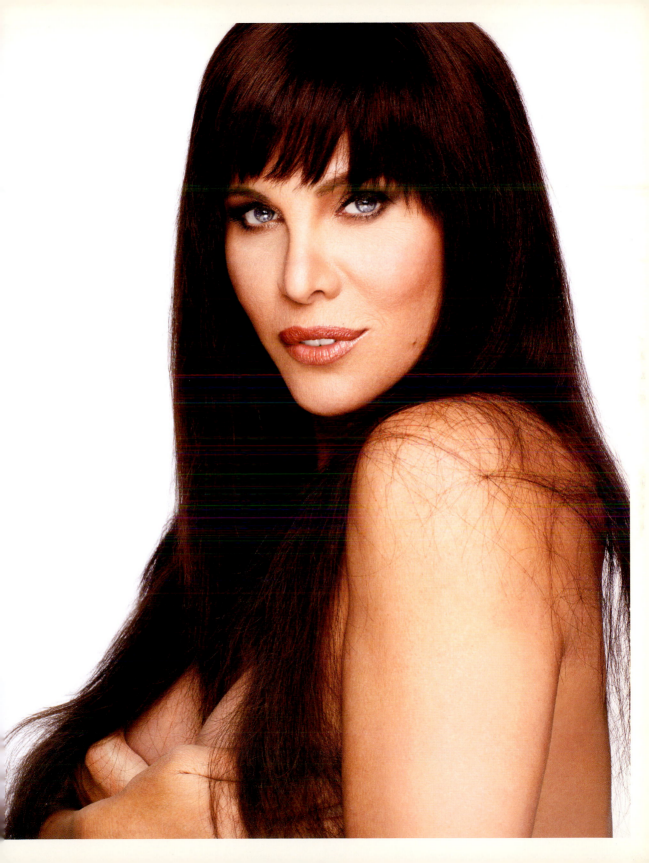

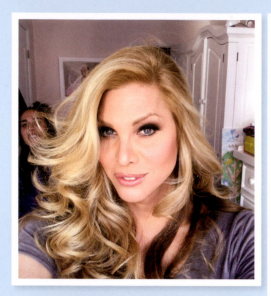
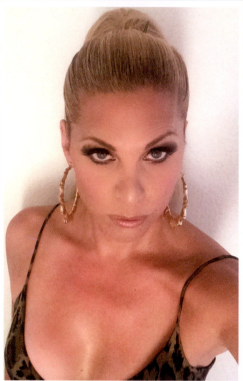
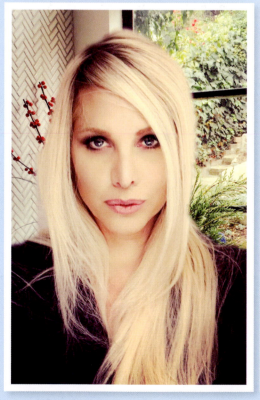
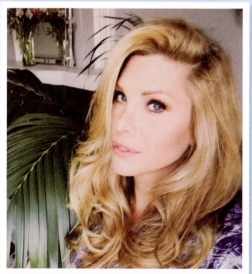

Some of my favorite hair looks.

- Use a larger round brush to achieve a nice volume and curve to your hair, especially when framing hair toward your face.
- For a softer, wispier curl, using a curling iron. Wrap large sections of your hair around the barrel in ringlets; run your fingers through the curls to spread them out.
- Use some pomade or your favorite styling product to create movement and a "messy hair" look.

Luscious long hair tips:
- Side sweeps are the softest, most feminine look ever for long hair.
- Have more fun with color (mermaid hair is so cool; just remember that the more vibrant the color, the harder the upkeep over time and it is a multistep process).
- You can have longer hair if you're older, just don't braid it like the Swiss Miss girl if you're over the age of twelve; simply pull it back in a ponytail or have it cut to frame your face.
- Use a detangling spray to keep your lovely locks from turning dread.
- Get your brush wet before brushing your hair, or use a wet brush for styling.
- Condition only the ends of your hair if you just want to avoid split ends.
- Let your hair air-dry as much as possible.
- Shampoo every other day versus every single day—this allows the natural oils to keep your hair hydrated.
- Trim your ends at least every six weeks.
- Alternate styles to keep your hair from getting limp.

MAINSTREAM MANES

What kind of hair does your favorite celebrity have? Which celebrities share *your* hair type? If you're not sure, take a look through the pages of hairstyle magazines at your favorite salon; there are always celebrities in the pages of those magazines to serve as inspiration. Here are a few that tend to appear most frequently:

JULIA ROBERTS: I think every woman secretly wants her hair; her auburn look is most flattering.

RIHANNA AND HALLE BERRY: Best short pixie cuts ever. I mean ever. Their hairstyles always make their faces seem like sculptures.

BEYONCÉ: Long, flowing hair that's enhanced by weaves—the gifts that keep on giving to Bey and her alter ego, Sasha Fierce.

KIM KARDASHIAN: The very definition of sleek, black hair; even if she's going for the wet-and-wavy look, her hair is always perfect.

SARAH JESSICA PARKER: From her *Sex*

and the City days to today, SJP's lovely long locks have been her most talked-about feature. Whether it's straight or curly, her hair always looks so full and healthy.

BLAKE LIVELY: The quintessential California blonde, and a woman who knows how and when to do a sexy side sweep.

HAIR 911

Those celebrities are lucky women, because their stylists are on speed dial. But what about you? Who can you call when you need emergency help with your hair? Here are some quick troubleshooting tips to get you through the day, at least until your stylist can see you:

GLAM ON THE GO

Keep an extra brush, a hair tie, and a travel-sized spray in your bag or glove compartment so you can change your look while you're out and about. A travel-sized bottle of leave-in conditioner for your gym or beach bag is also a good way to be sure your hair is well prepared for any activity.

VICTORIA BECKHAM: Trendsetter who rocked short hair until recently opting for a shoulder-length style with honey blonde highlights. And she rocks that look, too.

GWEN STEFANI: Medium or long, platinum blonde has never looked this good since the days of Jean Harlow.

KATE MIDDLETON: Classic royal beauty, and seriously the ideal successor to Princess Diana in terms of style.

ELLEN DEGENERES: Textured and androgynous at its celebrity best; Ellen's hair seems to dance right along with her, celebrating her uniqueness.

YOU TRIED COLORING YOUR HAIR AT HOME AND CHOSE THE WRONG SHADE: If it's too light, you may be able to use a color that is one or two shades darker to bring it back to reality. Too dark, and you'll need to have a professional tone it down. Pull it up into a ponytail, bun, or hat until the pros can fix it.

YOU DISCOVERED THAT CUTTING YOUR OWN HAIR WAS A BAD IDEA: This happens so often with bangs in particular. If you cut them too short, try applying some gel to the ends for a spunkier look; wave your hand over your bangs and then spray them down so they don't stick out.

YOUR HAIR IS BREAKING OR FALLING

OUT: Most often, this is the result of medications, so check with your doctor to see if you can make a switch. If it's happening because your hair is too dry, then try an at-home oil treatment or a leave-in conditioner. Sometimes chlorine can be another culprit; condition your hair every time after swimming.

YOUR HAIR IS ALL FRIZZY AND FRAZ-

ZLED: Try Frizz Ease from John Frieda. It's the best OTC help for the frizzies, and you can get it in several formats: mousse, spray, serum, shampoo, and conditioner.

YOUR HAIR IS TOO OILY AND ITCHY:
Sometimes, the pH balance is off and your hair needs a different formula. Women with this issue find that when they switch to men's shampoo, the problem suddenly disappears. Give it a try, but go for unscented shampoo or you'll smell like your dad all day long.

BECOME A HAIR WHISPERER

I know it may sound strange, but sometimes you just need to listen to your hair every day, to see what it *wants* to do. If it seems to want to go wavy, then work with it by putting a little bit of mousse or hair spray into the mix and gently scrunching up the waves with your hands. If it seems to be having a straight, serious day, then get out your straightener and accommodate it. Curly hair can get a bit wild, so may need a little taming, unless you are also in a wild mood. Hair isn't alive in the same way you live and breathe, but it can have a mind of its own depending on the environment, hormones, and even your own mood. Work with it, and it will cooperate with you rather than work against you—and we've all had those days, right?

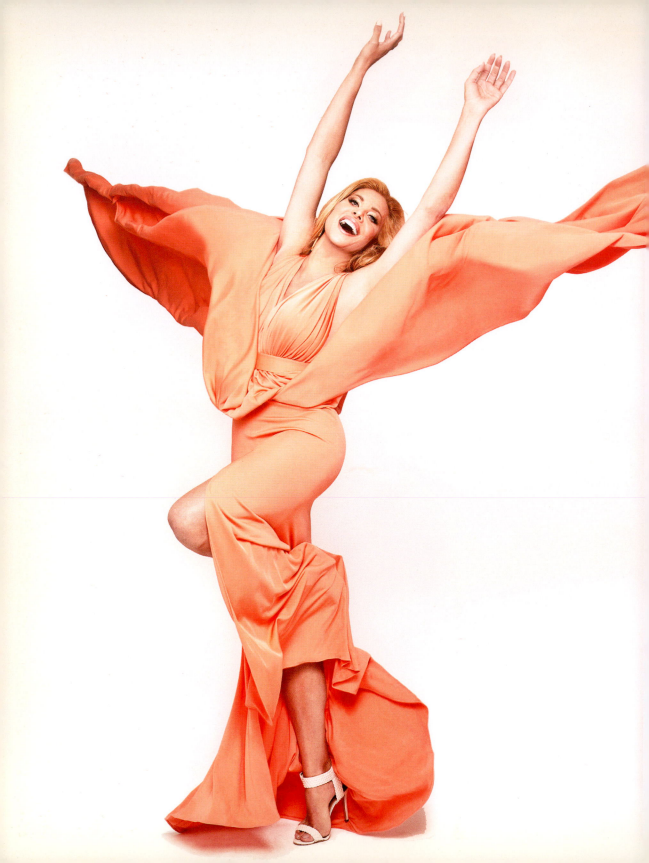

Part Three

Accentuating your True Self

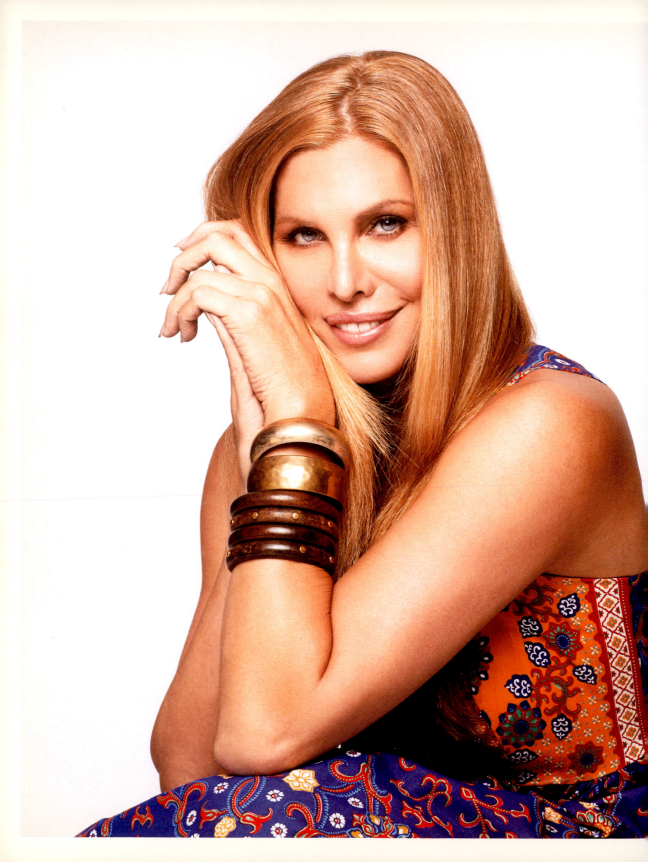

CHAPTER TEN:

WHO (AND WHAT) ARE YOU WEARING?

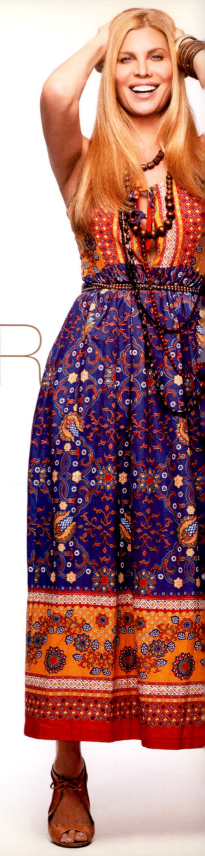

"GIVE A GIRL THE CORRECT FOOTWEAR AND SHE CAN CON- QUER THE WORLD."

—Bette Midler

B

elieve it or not, your clothing has a personality—and you can use it to your advantage. The trick is to figure out when you feel most yourself, and what you're wearing when you do. Don't know where to start? It's easy! Think about it this way: just about everyone has people in their life who see a piece of clothing in a store or magazine and say, "this is so *you*." Look in your closet, your Pinterest boards, or your guilty-pleasure mags. Find pieces others have said is the most "you." Then think, *are they really?* Trust your gut. Either way, there is an exciting fashion journey ahead of you—it could be to perfect what you already know is the most you, or to finally find out what is. It all begins and ends with shopping. That's the best part. And don't worry—I'll give you a few tips before you start hitting the racks.

WHAT'S YOUR BODY TYPE?

Some women are slender and petite; others are fuller and curvaceous. There are so many different ways for a body to be a body. No two are ever the same, and all of them are beautiful. That being said, each body deserves its own special fit—clothes that showcase its unique features instead of concealing them. Some women like to hide in their clothes. Insecurity can be expressed in fashion, too. Other women get distracted by the body type they *want* and try to showcase that body type instead of their own. You just have to remember that *every body* is beautiful, and there is no reason to hide.

I have more of a curvy body (unless I'm

in one of those superskinny moments in my life, which we all look back on and are super irritated with later), so I like to dress in clothes that are form-fitting, but not too tight.

Here are some specific tips for each of your lovely shapes:

'ROUND THE MIDDLE: If you are belly-dominant, choose clothes that fit you loosely around your middle (empire waists are great), but more tailored everywhere else (shoulders, arms, legs).

LIGHT TOP, HEAVIER BOTTOM: If your hips are your dominant feature, you need to avoid clingy materials like the plague. For pants, go with flare or wider-width; pair them with a form-fitting jacket, wider-neck blouse, or tailored cardigan. Dresses and skirts should be of stronger, nonclingy material, and give you an A-line look. If you want to wear skinny jeans, wear a top that is long and slightly tailored, to give you a more streamlined, A-line, or lightly tapered look. Don't be afraid of your curves—but keep it classy, girl.

GLAM ON THE GO

We all have that favorite outfit that makes us look and feel great. It doesn't matter who made it—it matters so much more how you make it express your true personality. The key is to find and wear outfits that *always* do that. Spend a little more on a great piece and less on filler. I have one caftan that makes me feel gorgeous and glam every time I put it on. It's so important to feel great about what you wear every day, so that you can carry that into living a confident and glowing life.

Choose slimming slacks or leggings, and match them up with a flowing blouse or tunic-style dress. This will focus attention on your slimmer portions. Also, don't be afraid of body-forming garment on nights out; my girlfriends and I have been gently cinching for years to add an extra bit of curviness.

PERFECT PROPORTIONS: Okay, so most of us already hate you for being an hourglass, because almost all of the clothing out there is secretly made for you. Still, you need to complement your curves with flowing wrap dresses, tailored blouses, and high-waisted slacks. A pencil skirt will work best for you.

SUPER STRAIGHT: You appear pencil-like and are likely tall as well, so go for a closer fit toward the middle and get looser as you move downward. You make the best use of the fitted jacket, as well as being able to pull off those fluffy poet blouses—and you are the only one who truly looks good in a flared or pleated skirt. Lucky you.

THE GOLDEN RULES

Let's get my two top rules when it comes to looking good in clothing out of the way:

1: FIND A GOOD TAILOR. If I wear a piece with no tailoring, I really can look boxy and square. The fact is, most often, you really need to tailor your clothes. Take in the waist, lift the hem, make it fit you as perfectly as possible. Almost no one fits 100 percent in every outfit they have, and that's why you need a good tailor in your life.

2: GET A STEAMER. Nothing looks worse than rumpled, ill-fitting fashion. That doesn't mean you have to save up for an expensive trip to the dry cleaner, though. You can do it all at home with your very own steamer. I got an industrial steamer that takes all of sixty seconds to steam up, and the wrinkles are gone. It's super easy. I

don't even know how to iron! The steamer only takes a few minutes and makes your clothes perfect again, especially after a good tailoring. Plus, there's no need to pinch pennies—there are cheap hand-held steamers at Walmart. So ditch what doesn't fit, fix what you need to fix, un-rumple what works, and let's go shopping.

LEARN BY LOOKING

Style isn't inherited, it's a skill. And we learn it from those around us. People walking down the street in New York City are dressed differently than people walking down the street in Los Angeles—and those same people were dressed even more differently a hundred years ago. Your style is impacted by where you are, who surrounds you, and what moves you. I learned a lot about my personal style by living in New York, a city filled with people of all races and sizes.

We have all met people with inherently great style and wonder, "How do they do it?" Confidence is the main ingredient. I don't believe in the words "age-appropriate." I believe in "confidence-appropriate" clothing, which means if your look makes sense as a good fit with your unique personality, go for it! If you're holding your own and pulling it off, more power to you. You have to learn to adapt, open yourself up to new possibilities, and never limit yourself to one look.

#THROWBACK-THRIFTING

Sometimes finding *your* look means borrowing ideas from the past that are still stylish today. Luckily, there are plenty of vintage stores in nearly every major city. I tend to go to places where the store owners already have a varying collection, and sometimes that may cost a little more, but you know you're getting authentic pieces in good condition.

Here's a fun way to help you learn the catalog of your local vintage stores: Back in my younger days, my girlfriend Lina and I used to play a game where we would get our monthly selection of *Vogue* or *Elle*, find a favorite look, and then go to the vintage store to see how well we could try and match it. Nine times out of ten we could do it. Not spot-on identically, mind you, but almost as perfect; the essence and the feel of that look were both there. Plus, a lot of times vintage clothes are made really well with great material (generally, if a piece of clothing is comprised of quality material, its cut will be better). Try it! You never know what hidden treasures might await you. Send me your results online at www.candiscayne.com. Don't overthink it. Use your instincts, and remember: less is more. You can dress up any outfit with a great jacket or fierce accessories. Adding layers is always easier than removing them, so don't feel the need to skimp on basics. Mix and match the old with the new; I always mix new clothes with a vintage piece so that I don't look like I came straight out of the '70s. Besides, blending the "then" and "now" pays homage to timeless fashion everywhere.

SAVVY SHOPPING

You have to pick your battles and spend money on classic pieces; these are the staples that you'll swap out and wear all the time, like:

- ❑ Five pairs of jeans (skinny dark, skinny light, boot-leg, straight-leg, and boyfriend jeans)
- ❑ Four tanks (two white, one gray, and one black)
- ❑ Four long-sleeved T-shirts (two white, one gray, and one black)
- ❑ Four short-sleeved T-shirts (two white, one gray, and one black)

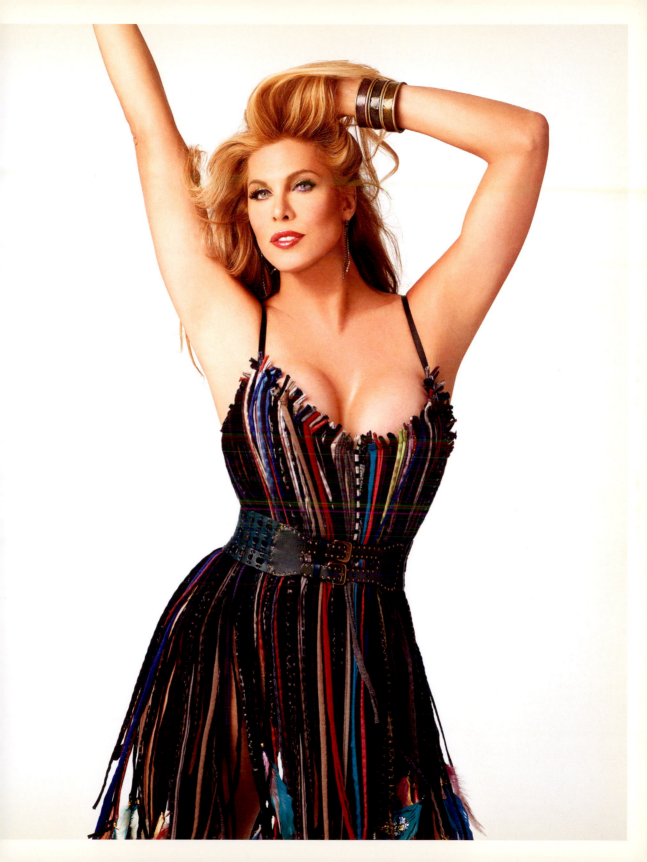

- One very white blouse (short- or long-sleeved, because it can be paired with a jacket)
- One casual T-shirt-style dress (these are easy to wear day or night with a simple change of accessories)
- One crew-necked and one cardigan sweater
- One sexy little black dress
- Two skirts (one dark, one light)
- One pair of black pants
- One denim jacket
- Colorful scarves
- Comfortable shoes (flat, ballet, tennis, or Oxfords)

Don't overthink it. Use your instincts, and remember: less is more.

- One pair of black heels (you can pack them and go easily from day to night looks, without even changing your jeans)
- A nice pair of boots (for dressing down in jeans, or making a casual dress a little more fun)
- Yoga pants, sweats, or soft casual clothes you can slip into (and out of) at any time of the day

Anything besides the basics are buys that you look and feel great in. Don't be afraid of color but be selective with pattern. Try,

try, try to buy things that are high-quality material—and are well made! The better the quality and presentation, the longer it'll last—and look great on you.

WARDROBE CLEANSING

A key ingredient to finding and maintaining your style personality is to keep your closet organized. My tip? I like to purge my closet a lot. I have clothes that I actually wear, and then I save pieces that have meaning, or are "Archive Pieces"—because

sometimes we get attached to certain things and can't let them go, even if they're never going to fit again. As for the rest of my closet, I have five sections: 1) Workout gear, 2) Day-casual, 3) Day-formal, 4) Evening-casual, and 5) Evening-formal. From there, I organize my wardrobe into colors, but you can do sleeve-length or divide it into even more numerical sections like size, if you like. Here's the bottom line: the easier it is to see what you *have*, the easier it will be to see what you *don't have*. And though it may seem daunting to create a wardrobe on a limited budget, having a clearer idea of what you do and don't need will make it that much easier. If you haven't looked at it or worn it in more than six months, time to purge. If you're like me, purging opens up a little space in your closet for your next piece—so saying good-bye opens you up to new fashion possibilities. Be brave and let it go!

GOT IT, FLAUNT IT?

One question a lot of women ask me is whether it's okay to flaunt what you've got. Listen, I've worked hard to get this body of mine, so of course I love to show it off whenever possible! I am in the public limelight often, so wearing low-cut gowns, or high-cut dresses that showcase my legs, or an off-shoulder classic sexy look, is perfect for me. But maybe you're a little more (or less) modest, preferring to selectively share your body's secret sweet spots. My only rules about that are: 1) Does it actually flatter your best parts, rather than cheapen your entire look, and 2) Is it expressing a natural extension of your personality to others?

So often, I see women (especially younger ones at the clubs) who really seem like they are doing cosplay as streetwalkers. (Now, don't get me wrong—I've worn a short dress or two in my life—but it's how you wear them that matters.) It's like they don't have the confidence in who they are to lead with their inner shine—so they resort to uncomfortably low-cut blouses and shoes they can barely walk in sober, let alone after a few drinks. It's one thing if you're comfortable like that, day or night, but another thing altogether if it's about pretending to be more available, more outgoing, than you are in your actual life. There's a saying that the people who do the best at job interviews are the ones who are best at being themselves—and that's just as true when you are out on the town, presenting yourself to potential partners. Don't show up in your gym clothes, but do wear clothes that fit who you really are at this moment in time—and don't be afraid to shine from the inside out.

On the flip side, what if you are too conservative for your own good? If you prefer to stay buttoned up all the time, you need a fashion intervention just as much as the girl who's trying to look like Nicki Minaj. A look that plays it too safe can age you faster than a week in the sun. Unless you actually are a librarian, you don't want to look like one, right? The best way to update your wardrobe is to check it first for all of the classic pieces (listed on page 148–150)—move those to one side of your closet, and everything else to the other. Grab a best friend, someone who can honestly assess

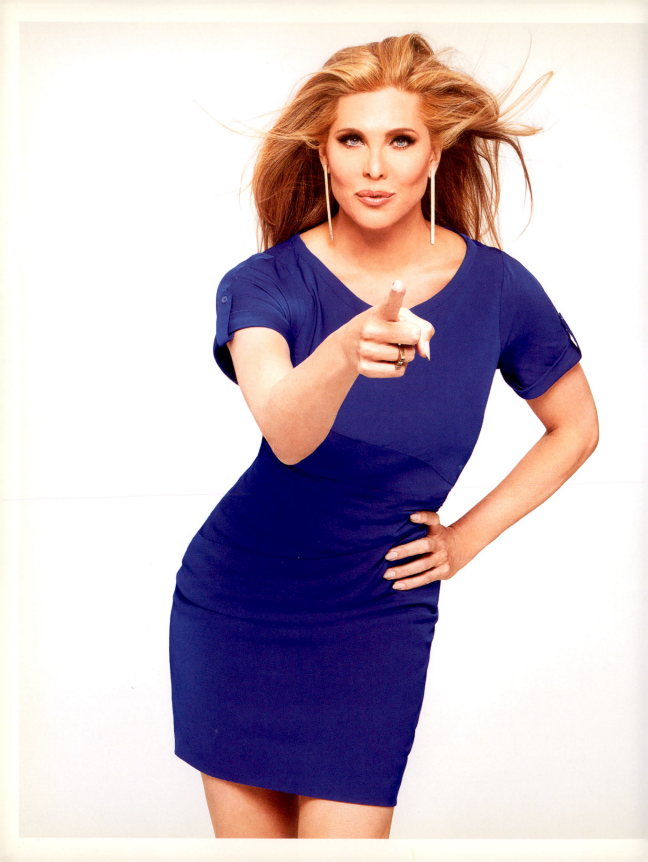

what's left and support you in the drive to the Goodwill drop-off bin. You need the pieces that are just taking up space in your closet out of your life as soon as possible, so you can focus on enhancing, supplementing, and updating all of your classic looks.

WHAT LIES BENEATH

We've talked about the major pieces you'll need to keep your wardrobe timeless and pretty—but what about what's underneath it

buy yourself one size slightly larger than your actual size, because then you will not have the bulging panty lines that so many of our ill-informed sisters suffer through (and make others witness to) on a daily basis. Do not lie to yourself about your true size, but instead focus on comfort first, looks second. You can definitely buy yourself lovely lacies, but make sure they don't look like lovely pasties (unless you're going for a burlesque look, which of course is fine).

From a hygiene standpoint, you'll want to stick with a cotton crotch if possible, even if you're into thongs. These harbor less

Style isn't inherited, it's a skill.
And we learn it from those around us.

all? Often, we get so wrapped up in spending our money on the outside appearance, and then are forced to go cheap on the undergarments. But that works, right? In a word, no. Quality does count. Personally, I wear Hanky Pankys, mostly because of the way they fit my body, with no visible panty lines.

The number-one rule about underwear is that it needs to fit you correctly. How many times have you been in a locker room at the gym and seen a plus-sized woman trying to stuff herself into panties she's probably had since she was twelve? No, girlfriend. No way. Honor your size, and, in fact, even

of the nasty bacteria that can wreak havoc on your private parts—so, ladies, keep it clean while you're putting on your Victoria's Secrets.

What about bras? There are two kinds that one should have in their wardrobe: two T-shirt bras and two or more sexy lace bras in black and nude. If you're not sure what size to buy, get a true bra fitting from a professional—it's a free service available at most department stores.

Even if no one ever sees them, I find that I feel sexy and empowered with the right kind of undergarments. It'll do the same for you!

SHOE ADDICTS UNITE

Shoes, glorious shoes! We all have a little bit of Imelda Marcos in us, don't we? But honestly, how do you know which ones are the perfect fit for your princess feet? Which ones flatter while also making your heart flutter?

Let's start with fit. Have your feet measured by an actual shoe sales person. Even if you think you've always been a perfect size 7, your feet can change over time (especially due to hormones or having kids). By making sure you know your size, you can better ensure that you won't wind up with too much space in your heels, or too little space in the toes of your shoes. This will help you to walk better, too, because you will be in better balance. There's nothing more painful than seeing a woman whose feet are swollen and painful from trying to walk in shoes that are really too small (or too high in the heel for comfort). Stilettos are sexy, but only if they are a good fit, and only if you can actually walk in them without using your partner as a crutch. If you're wobbling, you won't come across as your confident, gorgeous self.

For heels, three inches is a comfortable height—one that most women can achieve without pinching, slipping, wobbling, or falling forward. If you want to go higher, that's fine—just be sure you can walk safely and confidently.

When I'm shopping for heels, I try to find genuine leather shoes and soles. They may be a bit more expensive, but usually are so much better for your feet. I do the move test: I grab the sole with one hand and the heel with another, to see how much movement there is; if it's stiff as a board, I pass, because our feet move when they walk, so they need shoes that give a little.

Not all women can wear flats—especially those with fallen arches or slender heels. Those with slender heels tend to slip right out of them, so if you're one of these ladies, you'll either need to include a heel insert or wear flats with laces instead. Ballet flats are so great to keep around for those who can wear them, though, because you can toss them into your car or bag when going from office to a night on the town—and then you can put them back on for the ride home.

Sandals can be of any height or style, as long as they complement whatever you're wearing. Gladiators that go up to your knee paired with a soft, lace summer dress aren't an ideal choice—but a pair of dressy flip-flops (not cheap beach ones) or leather strappy sandals would look great. The softer the look, the softer the shoe. Simple enough?

One more thing: for athletic shoes, you

need to go one half size to one whole size larger, because your feet will swell a bit with exercise (and you're likely wearing thicker socks). Buy separate pairs for walking, running, or workouts—you need the right shoe for each type of exercise, because believe it or not, they are built differently on purpose. It's not a one-size-fits-all thing.

What are your fashion rules?

PATRICIA FIELD:
"Choose one-of-a-kind pieces. Anything in silk and cashmere."

SCOTT BARNES:
"Know your audience; wear the proper dress to the proper event. Also, figure out your basic 'little black dress' look (i.e., your signature style); you can always embellish from there. It should not be an exercise in terror every time you go to get ready."

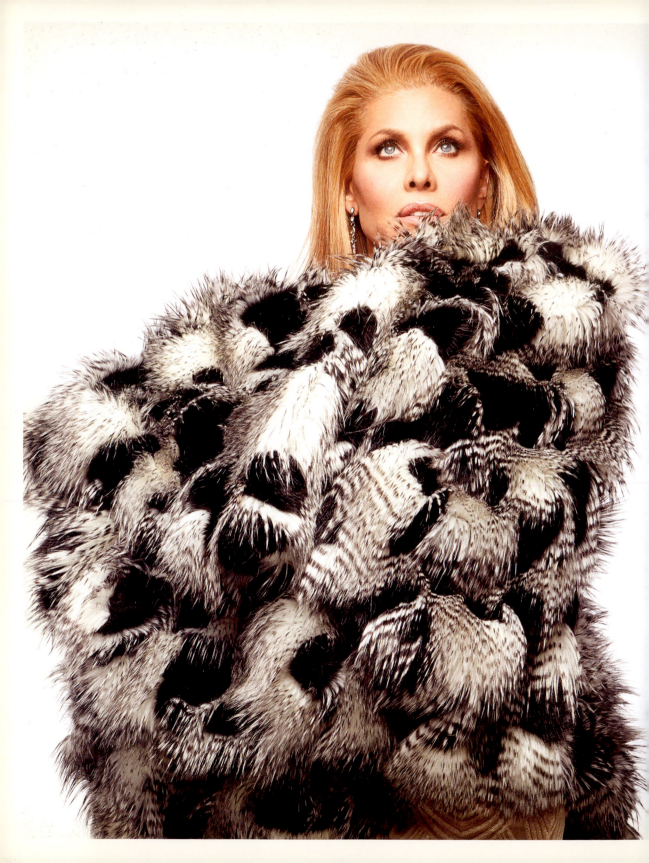

CHAPTER ELEVEN:

DELICIOUS DÉCOR

"STYLE IS A WAY TO SAY WHO YOU ARE WITHOUT HAVING TO SPEAK."

—Rachel Zoe

hen it comes to accessories, I definitely go for a less-is-more approach. That's my personal preference, but it really is something that you have to decide based on trial and error. Sometimes big statement pieces work for people—other times, small and subtle accessories are the go-to. I have friends who love chunky, hefty jewelry and it looks great on them. Don't be discouraged if those types of pieces don't work right for you. The most important thing to remember is that you are the star of the show, not the accessories. Don't let your jewelry wear you. Even if I'm wearing an eight-pound necklace, it should be the star of the *outfit*—not of *me*. Fashion is supposed to showcase, not overwhelm. It can be easy to get carried away when it comes to sparkles and glitter, so remember what Coco Chanel said: "Before you leave the house, look in the mirror and remove one accessory." Tough love from Coco, but she may be right. Don't overdo a good thing. The question is, how do you know when it's a good thing? Let's take a look in our jewelry boxes and find out.

BOLD JEWELRY STATEMENTS

There are many ways to build a nice, diverse collection of jewelry over the years.

As for me? I had an earring stalker. I know it sounds scary, but it was actually kind of funny. A box would show up at my house every so often with tons of earrings—every type you could imagine—and this went on for years. In fact, to this day I never learned who it was and how they got my address (which is the scary part). Over time I realize that no matter how many pieces I had, I always went back to a handful of favorites.

So, since that's not how all of you are going to build your earring collections, hitting up thrift stores and places like T.J. Maxx and Marshall's will enable you to create your own collection in a much less

cool, chunky vintage necklace, or an extra-long, dangly set of earrings. Sometimes all it takes is a fun statement piece to take an outfit to the next level.

Adding fun pieces to your outfits isn't where the accessorizing ends: I get crafty about displaying them. I got one side of an old dog cage and screwed it to the wall—it's about 3 x 3 and the perfect way to hang

CHANNELING YOUR INNER FAIRY GLAM-MOTHER

We all have those moments in life where we're invited for a last-minute get-to-gether, or for some impromptu drinks after work. When that happens, we don't have time to run home and entirely change our outfit—and no one realistically keeps a handy-dandy set of emergency party clothes in their trunk. The idea is to have a few tricks up your sleeve that can help turn your everyday casualwear into some evening fun at the last minute. It's easier than you think, because all it takes is a few accessories in the right place at the right time. That's the great thing about accessories. If you're wearing a pair of jeans and tank during the day and you want to wear the same outfit for evening, you just need four simple things: a great lipstick, a chunky necklace or earrings, a cute jacket, and a pair of heels or dressier shoes. Then, abracadabra! You're all glammed up for the night. No magic necessary—just a few trendy pieces you could keep in your car or in your office, and you'll be ready for whenever nightlife calls.

creepy way. Go for pieces that are flexible and will match a lot of your wardrobe, and then go for some that are different than anything you already have, even if they won't match much. When it comes to jewelry, I say go bold. Everyone should have a couple of statement pieces in their arsenal, like a

your earrings so that you can see them easily. Who says your jewelry can't *always* be on display, especially in your own house? Take a look on Pinterest to see all the fun and simple DIY home jewelry displays. Give some a try, and send me pics. Let's be real, our walls deserve to be just as glam as us.

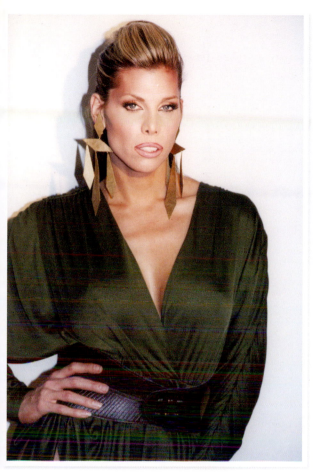
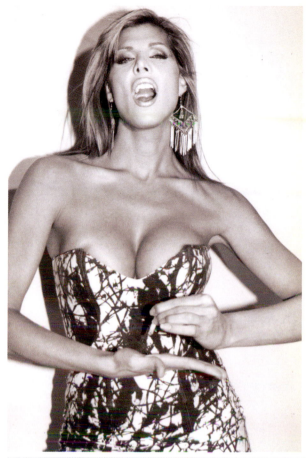

LEFT: Huge earrings can add drama and dimension to your look.

RIGHT: Some earrings are such a strong focal point, they require no other jewelry.

DIAMONDS IN THE ROUGH

"So, Candis," you say, "where can we possibly find these cool statement pieces you keep talking about?" A lot of the time, those vintage stores we talked about last chapter have jewelry counters with tons of awesome pieces! You really just have to do a little digging at your local thrift stores and you won't be disappointed. Go for something bold and one-of-a-kind—something you definitely can't find at any other popular retail hotspot. Secondhand and even antique stores are your best bet. Don't be discouraged by a little surface dirt, either: pick up a gentle jewelry cleaner at Target or Walmart, and you'll be surprised at how quickly a piece can transform. We're not all experts at this kind of #throwbackthrifting, though, so here are some quick dos and don'ts for shopping vintage or antique jewelry:

DO: Go for personality, charm, and quality. You're looking for statement pieces, so really go out of your comfort zone and get something that just makes you say "Wow!" It's supposed to stand out in a fun and unique way, so don't be afraid of getting too "out there" with it. Be sure that it's decent enough quality, though, before you toss it in your cart.

DON'T: Take home pieces that are too rusted, visibly missing any stones or gems, tangled beyond hope, or have any other super-glaring blemishes. Some light cleaning and upkeep is totally reasonable for a purchase like this, but if you have to go full-on jewelry ER, then the piece may not be worth the investment.

Have fun but be cautious, and I guarantee you'll find some one-of-a-kind head-turners that'll perfectly accessorize to your favorite outfits.

BODY ART

"I am a canvas of my experiences," says tattoo artist Kat Von D. "My story is etched in lines and shading, and you can read it on my arms, my legs, my shoulders, and my stomach." We've all totally had starry eyes for people like Kat Von D before, am I right, ladies? Some of us have tattoos, some of us are trying to muster the courage to get them, and some of us are a little too intimidated by the permanence of a tattoo to *really* get starry-eyed. Ditto for piercings. Body mods can be totally scary. But they're also an integral part of fashion, style, and self-expression. Our mods become part of us.

In 1992, I decided to get a belly piercing. I had no tattoos or piercings and I thought it would be cute (and, at the time, almost no one had one). I still have it. I love it, and it's just a part of me now. I almost feel naked without it. It was a personal choice of my style, so I say if you want a piercing or tattoo, get it. Just make sure it's for you and that you love it. Remember, in the case of a tattoo it is quite permanent, so choose wisely—going for your boyfriend or girlfriend's name isn't always the best idea! Draw the tattoo on yourself in permanent marker for a few weeks to see if you really like it. Get it in henna first. Really, really make sure that whatever it is you're adding to your body is for you and you alone. It's your body and your decision, so make sure you listen to your heart and don't let yourself get pressured into something that isn't exactly what you want. Do research on your tattoo and piercing parlor options—meet with the artists, get to know their style, shop around. Tattoos and other body mods are special, intimate, and oftentimes eternal expressions of you. Make sure they're as perfect as their "canvas" before they get painted on for good!

COMPLEMENTING YOUR CAPSULE WARDROBE

One of the trendiest closet organization techniques is called the capsule wardrobe, and I'm going to tell you how to accessorize the basic fashion version we created in the last chapter (page 148–150). It's super simple, and it's just the kind of process that will help you really get to know your closet and your own personal style inside and out.

By the way, the term "capsule wardrobe," coined by Susie Faux in the 1970s, is really just a fancy name for a minimalist closet made up of a few basic pieces paired with a seasonal rotation of accessories. It enables you to hand-pick a small, stock wardrobe based on your body type, complexion, and personality, leaving you plenty of room year-round to add new purchases of fun color and fabric schemes when the seasons change, and you find yourself in need of a cardigan instead of a sundress.

Are you sold yet? Here are a few steps to get you started toward your own stylish and flexible accessory portion of the capsule wardrobe. Not coincidentally, it begins with the same kind of closet purge we did in the previous chapter:

- Go through your closet and pull out every bag, belt, scarf, and piece of jewelry that you haven't used in the past year—and you're only allowed a couple of exceptions based on sentimentality!
- Look at what's left and pull out the things you hardly ever wear anymore. Whether they're not your style, or they're not as "vogue" as they used to be, if you're not wearing them as accessories, then they're liable to become accessories to "fashion crimes."
- Make sure all that remains are the accessories you wear regularly, and that you look and feel great in.
- Bag up the castaways and take them to your nearest donation center—even if they didn't make the cut for your closet, they're bound to make it for someone else's!

There, didn't that feel as great as the clothing purge? It's always healthy to go through purges like this at least once a year. It's easy to end up with an overcrowded closet, so taking the time to pare it down is both necessary and totally cathartic. The key is to start with only the accessory essentials in your closet. So, what counts as essentials? Let's make a list of what you'll need:

- ❏ Two pairs of black or brown boots (one ankle-length, one higher—even thigh-high if you'd like)
- ❏ One pair of black or neutral ballet flats
- ❏ One pair of high heels
- ❏ One pair of casual shoes
- ❏ One pair of workout shoes
- ❏ Four purses (one classic style, one boho, one travel, and one "statement" such as a designer or artist bag)
- ❏ One clutch (for evening wear)
- ❏ One tote bag (beach or travel)
- ❏ One raincoat
- ❏ One winter coat
- ❏ Three belts (one black, one brown, and one multicolored or scarf-like belt)

How much did you already have? I'll bet you're off to a great start. When you have the essentials, mixing and matching scarves, jewelry, shoes, and accessories will become second nature. Imagine how many different combinations of outfits you could put together in just one week with only the few accessories listed above—and now imagine adding some fun seasonal pieces to the mix! The hardest part about maintaining a totally complete capsule wardrobe is sticking to the basics and only adding a few seasonal must-haves: otherwise, your closet will end up just as full as before the purge. It's tricky, but it can be done, and you'll feel great for doing it. To help you stay on task, here are some season-by-season suggestions to navigating those trendy temptations:

FOR FALL: Try to limit yourself to only one infinity scarf and one cardigan. Remember: you already have boots, so don't even think about stepping foot in the shoe store. I know there are tons of supercute fall items out at shoe stores, but stop and ask yourself, "Do I really need a new pair of boots?" Unless the answer is yes, stick to some fun fall-patterned flannels or sweaters as your new fall buys.

FOR WINTER: You'll definitely need your token ugly Christmas sweater, right? (Just kidding.) Seriously, go for one elegant holiday party dress and you'll be all set.

FOR SPRING: Pick up one or two flirty sundresses—with a face-defining straw hat and dramatic sunglasses. Your summer body will thank you for the exposure in all the right places!

FOR SUMMER: The dreaded bathing suit season. Don't put so much pressure on yourself. Find a fun swimsuit that you feel great in and call it a day. Use the buddy system and go shopping with a girlfriend if you feel like you need the emotional support. Go to a juice bar to celebrate afterward.

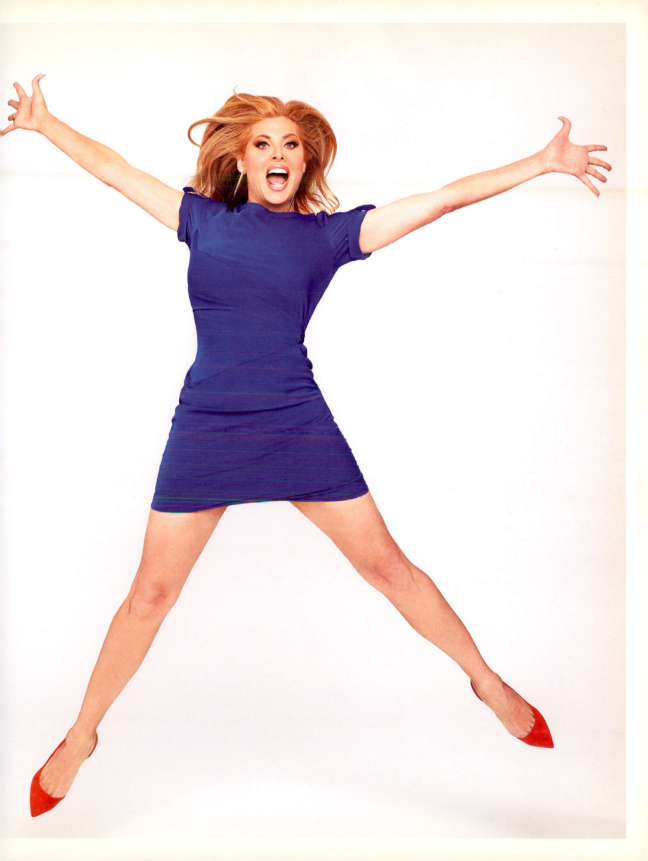

Believe it or not, these are all the seasonal clothes and accessories you really need. Before your seasonal additions, that's a modest thirty-eight-piece wardrobe. After you throw in a couple flannels, sweaters, dresses, and swimsuits, your overall wardrobe shouldn't exceed forty-five items (not counting jewelry), and that's being generous. Be accountable—don't overspend or overstock. You honestly don't need more than you already have. Mix and match, and get creative! You are already blessed with everything you need to be your truest, most stylish self.

BAGGIN' IT

When it comes to arm-candy, stick with quality over quantity—and practicality, first and foremost. A lovely clutch that is too small to carry your most important portable possessions is not going to be a great buy because you simply won't use it as often as larger, more accommodating bags. When you go shopping for a new bag, take the wallet you plan to use with it, as well as any other go-to accessories (i.e., sunglasses, lip gloss, etc.), and literally try on the bag in the store. So few women do this, and yet you wouldn't just buy a pair of shoes without trying them on first! Make sure the bag meets the need first, then choose a style or color that best matches or complements the look you're perfecting. It doesn't need to match your shoes 100 percent, as it did in your mom's day; you can add interest and dimension to your look with an appealing (yet still practical) bag, as long as it does not become the only focal point.

I say have fun with the look, color, and

What's your best accessory advice?

PATRICIA FIELD:
"When it comes to accessories, focus on belts, hats, and personally meaningful jewelry. Those really help define your style in a way that is unique from everyone else."

JENNIFER RADE:
"Beware of shorter, thicker necklaces, as they can cut your shape in an unflattering way."

SCOTT BARNES:
"Nobody loves a 'trendy Wendy.' Wearing every trend at once makes you a walking trend report. Remember, trends are there to draw inspiration from, so use a little piece here or there, not all at once."

woven materials in the bags you choose—just don't wear one that hangs so long on your body that you look like you're going to a Grateful Dead tribute concert. Unless, of course, you are actually going to one. Conversely, don't wear bags that are too short under the arm, especially if you have larger arms or a curvier body. In these cases, you'll look like you've stuffed a sausage roll under your arm.

At home, one cool way to keep your best bags visible is to hang them on the walls of your closet as works of art (and aren't most of the really sweet ones?). This way, you can see them pretty much every day, making it easier to choose one to switch off for another while keeping your closet "gallery" more visually interesting. I've seen several walls that only contain vintage purses, too. Isn't that a fun idea?

WELCOME TO THE WORKING WEEK

So, how can you best accessorize yourself for an entire week, now that you've got your closet game down? Particularly for work, the best thing to do is wear your more conservative jewelry during the daytime, with maybe one good signature piece (like a one-of-a-kind item from a jewelry artist).

Too many times, women overaccessorize for what they perceive to be a "power" look, when really it is just a bit overpowering. As I've said, less is more, and it's all about quality. You don't want to look like Madonna in the '80s if you're trying to put your best foot forward in this decade. One good scarf, and one exciting, eye-catching signature piece, for just a few days and you have what you need to mix and match with just about every outfit all week long.

A good strand of pearls can be part of a power look, too, and are easy to pair up with just about any outfit, day or night. The great thing about pearls is you can dress up a look with them by their simple addition—but they can also be worn with a blouse, denim jacket, and flowing skirt with some cowboy boots for a more casual elegance.

A good rule of thumb for earrings and bracelets is to start small for earlier in the day, and work your way out to larger, fascinating pieces for evening wear. I keep some pieces in a bag for easier day-to-night transition. (Remember: Stuff an emergency accessory pack in your glove compartment for those more spontaneous nights out!)

The key is to have a good mix of silver, gold, and colorful accessories—each with the capability of playing your look up or down, depending on where you are and what you are doing throughout the day.

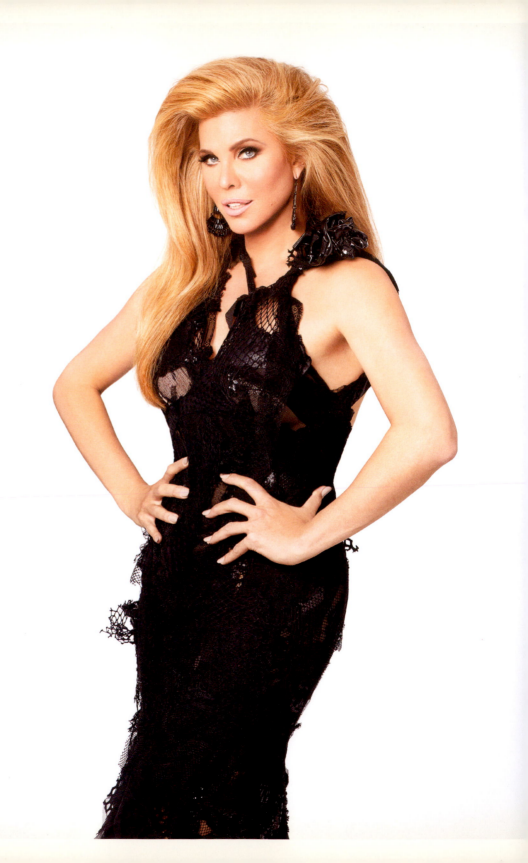

CHAPTER TWELVE

PUTTING THE BEST YOU FORWARD

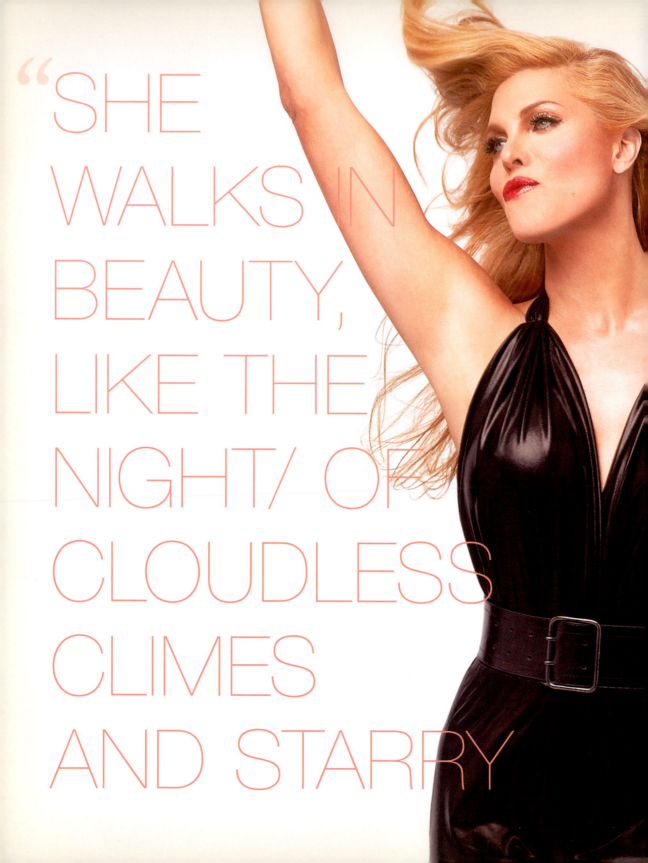

"SHE WALKS IN BEAUTY, LIKE THE NIGHT/ OF CLOUDLESS CLIMES AND STARRY

SKIES;/ AND ALL THAT'S BEST OF DARK AND BRIGHT/ MEET IN HER ASPECT AND HER EYES."

—Lord Byron, George Gordon

To me, to "walk in beauty" means to walk through life with joy, elegance, compassion, and confidence—and to live your life as your authentic self. Confidence is 9/10 of the law. We're instantly attracted to anyone who has confidence; it comes from just knowing that you're always in the right place at the right time— and knowing that you're enough. And it's no secret that nowadays, that can be really hard.

A lot of times we don't value ourselves, and we let others dictate what we believe, what we like, and who we are. We let people run over us, and sometimes we feel the need to run over others. We try to out-twirl or out-flirt another girl. Or we try to "blend in." We try to have ambition, but not too much. But this is no way to live. We should live this life as the best "us" we can, which, to me, *is* glamorous. We are enough. I watch all the time as women wait for a man or woman or relationship, thinking that if they are able to find this person, *then* they will feel whole, or confident, or glamorous. I say, find yourself and what makes you feel whole on your own, and then find a partner who is worthy of your greatness and wholeness. Wait for what's right. A lot of times women settle for less than they deserve because their entire lives, they have been made to feel by the media, by their parents, and by society that they are "less than." It's time to really realize that we are *not*.

Confidence is not putting people down, or having an over-inflated ego. You can be confident and gracious at the same time. I see some people who appear confident on the surface but underneath are just demeaning divas, which, to me, is not only a lack of confidence but also a bigger sign of insecurity. While you're walking in beauty, the bottom line is to never forget your own value and, just as important, always remember everyone else's, too.

BEING YOUR OWN FEARLESS LEADER

What is fearlessness? Well, the first time I saw fearlessness was when my mom joined a basketball team when I was probably five or six, and the players were all men—they begrudgingly allowed her to play after weeks of sitting on the sidelines, only to run circles around the competition. She would bring me to the games sometimes and I would watch in awe. For myself, I think I found it in high school. My junior year, I was sent to Los Angeles to go to school and was kicked out because I was effeminate and they thought I was gay. After that I realized that the world was going to treat me a certain way, so I had to face it head-on with confidence or I'd be swallowed up. To me, that's what fearlessness is: facing adversity head-on, with confidence. Life isn't easy, we all know this. So that's why we need to spend as much time as we can be building ourselves and one another other up!

But building confidence is easier said than done. Sometimes it takes everything we've got just to get out of bed in the morning, let alone be happy about it. So, let's try and make it simple. Here is a supereasy checklist to help your daily journey toward self-love. Try to do each one of these things on the list once a day! You'd be surprised

at how much better you'll feel if you turn these actions into habits:

- Tell yourself you're gorgeous. I mean it. Stand in front of the mirror, look yourself in the eye, and say it until you believe it.
- Do something that energizes you. Go to the gym, do yoga, go for a walk. The more you move around and get physical, the better you'll feel. It's those fun little things called "endorphins" that come out to play whenever you start shaking your groove-thang. Trust me, you'll get addicted to them once you show them you mean business.
- Drink lots of water. Keeping hydrated helps you stay healthy and on point.
- Have some "me" time. Set aside some time during the day to spend with yourself. Relax and mingle with your thoughts. Odds are you're better company than you think, and you deserve to take a second to appreciate yourself. Take a luxury bath, give yourself a mani/pedi, or go people-watch at Starbucks.
- Present the best "you" possible, which means, stay positive, upbeat, and engaged. Dress for success and put on your game face, because you should always be ready to rock 'n' roll.

There, not so hard, right? Just five quick steps to add to your daily routine that will really help you grow confidence and minimize insecurity. You've got to learn to create a total sensory experience for others—and that includes the scent you leave behind.

FRAGRANCE AS A FINISHING TOUCH

Part of putting the best "you" forward is putting *all* of you forward. That means outfits, accessories, makeup, and even how you smell to others. That's right, perfume is just as integral to your style as your clothes. So, what's your "signature scent"? I like mine a bit earthy, musky, and floral. My absolute favorite is "Wish" by Chopard, with Hermès as a close second. They just seem to work with my chemistry for a knockout scent. But I'm Italian and feisty, so while these work for me, they may not work for everyone. Decide what kind of scent you are by asking friends or doing research online, but always test them out before you make a purchase. Think about a smell that compliments you but doesn't overpower. If you want a fresh, clean smell go with a citrus or linen—that's the safest bet, for starters. Head to your local department store or Bath & Body Works and start spritzing away until you really connect with a scent. T.J. Maxx also has a huge selection of brand-name perfumes for affordable prices. Just remember, the way you smell plays a huge part in your first impression, as well as the lasting memory you leave, so always make it a point to smell as radiant as you look! Here's a handy guide to getting started on the quest for your signature scent:

FLORAL: Ah, the belle of the ball with the timeless style. If you love florals, odds are you're the old-fashioned gal of your squad with a soft spot for tender, classic romance.

MUSK: You might have been in your high school drama club, and Halloween might be your favorite holiday. If you like mature, dramatic scents, then musk might be your new go-to.

FRUITY: You're the fun, flirty girl of the bunch who is outgoing, trendy, and totally fashion-savvy, right? Then the fruity scent definitely has your name written all over it.

CITRUS: If you're drawn to the citrus scents, you may identify as a modern go-getter, leader, or jetsetter. Women who pick this scent are always the first out of bed in the morning with a smile on their face, ready to take on the world.

SWEET AND SPICY: You're sexy and you know it. Confidence is your middle name and everyone wants your number. More like sugar, spice, and everything *classy*, am I right?

POWDER AND LINEN: Between work-out sessions and trips to the juice bar, do you even have time to shop for perfume? Let me make it easy for you—you love smelling fresh, clean, and rejuvenated, just like you stepped straight out of a steaming hot shower, right?

PRESENTING YOUR BEST SELFIE

Okay, now that you are all put together, how are you going to present yourself to the rest of the world visually? With the power of the Internet nowadays, making a good impression online is just as critical as making one offline. It's already stressful enough trying to be your best self in real life—but what about from behind the screen? I find myself being more drawn to people who are easy and can laugh at themselves and not take everything so seriously. When you're online, it's so important to be yourself and let your inner radiance shine. These days, so much happens online. You can score dates or job interviews; you can become a vlogging sensation or a saleswoman. The world is truly at your fingertips every time you log in. So, how do you make the best of it? First things first, you're going to need a killer profile-pic. Whether it's for Facebook, LinkedIn, YouTube, Twitter, or OkCupid, you'll want to look your best. But taking selfies isn't as easy as it seems. Here's some advice on how to up your selfie game:

- Always shoot for natural lighting. Stand by the window, by the door, or just, you know, go outside (if you do go outside, make sure you are blocking the sun so it doesn't harshen the quality of your pic). Natural light highlights your face in all the right places and will leave you glowing. Overhead lighting when taking a selfie is horrible, so avoid it.

The world is truly at your fingertips every time you log in.

- For mirror selfies, always make sure the light isn't coming from behind. You want the light to be coming from above or in front of you, ideally. If you're backlit, you'll end up looking like a shadow.
- Don't put the camera too high up, but rather put it closer to your face. Keep your chin down to elongate your face and give it a more elegant appearance.
- Think about what's in the background of your selfie. Even if your face looks totes adorbs, odds are it won't be enough to distract from the pile of dirty laundry behind you!

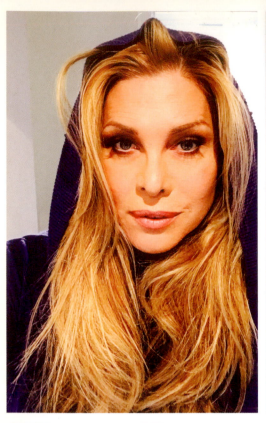
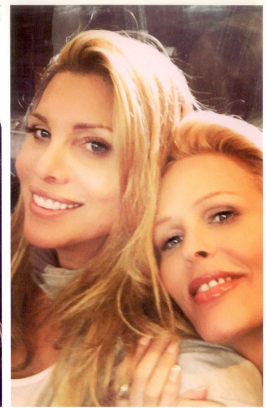
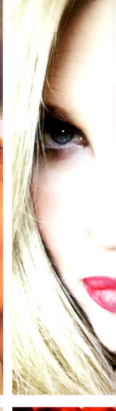
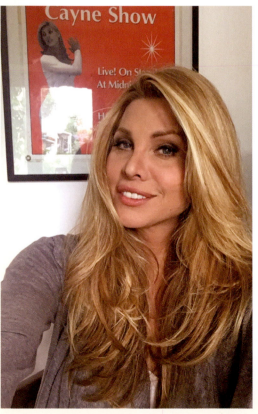
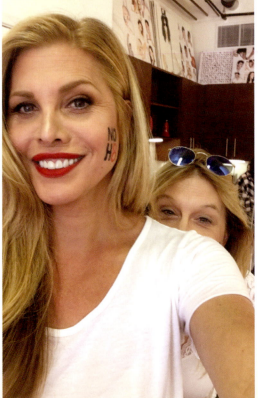
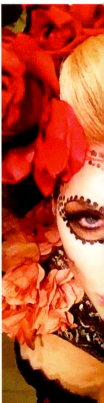

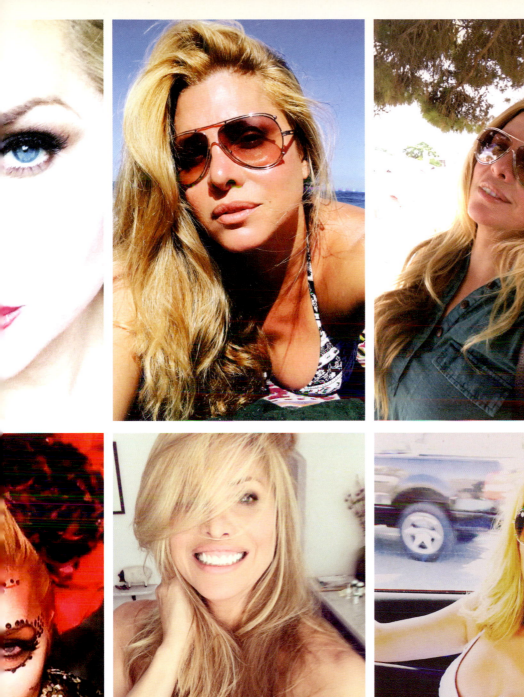
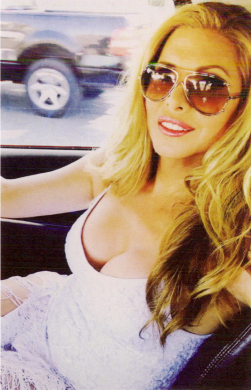

- Try out some fun angles. Don't always put your face in the middle or in one corner. Explore and get creative!
- If you're really hardcore into your Internet game, you may want to consider investing in a nice, digital camera rather than a cell phone.

LIGHTS, CAMERAS, ACTION!

Now that we've got selfies covered, let's take it a step further—into vlogging. How do you start vlogging, and what do you need? Here's my advice:

- Do your homework. Get to know the current vloggers out there and pick your favorites. What do they talk about, and how do they script their posts? There's all kinds of vlogging to be done—shopping, makeup, gossip, DIY crafting—find your niche and go for it.
- Invest in some basic vlogging gear. A camera, a tripod, and, of course, a set. Where are you going to film, what does it say about you, and how does it compliment your topics?
- Decorate your filming area the same way you'd decorate yourself for a good first impression.
- Write a script or an outline to help you stay on topic. Rehearse, rehearse, rehearse!
- Engage your audience by asking questions (they can leave their answers in your comments section) and using props. If you're vlogging about your latest shopping haul, using your purchases as "props" will be super easy, for example.
- Use some fun musical underscoring, when applicable, with a video editing program (most laptops these days come with a simple video editor, so be sure to read up on which programs come with your devices).
- Don't exceed five or six minutes in length. People don't have an elastic attention span, so make sure to say what you need to say and wrap it up. Leave your viewers wanting more!
- Be yourself. That's the most important advice I can give you. No two people are the same, and everyone has something unique and fun to offer, especially when it comes to vlogging. Find what makes you tick and show the virtual world!

LOOKIN' FOR LOVE

Let's review: not only can you now take jaw-dropping selfies, but you're also super vlogging-savvy and are probably off to becoming the next hottest YouTube sensation. What can't you do, girl? Time to move

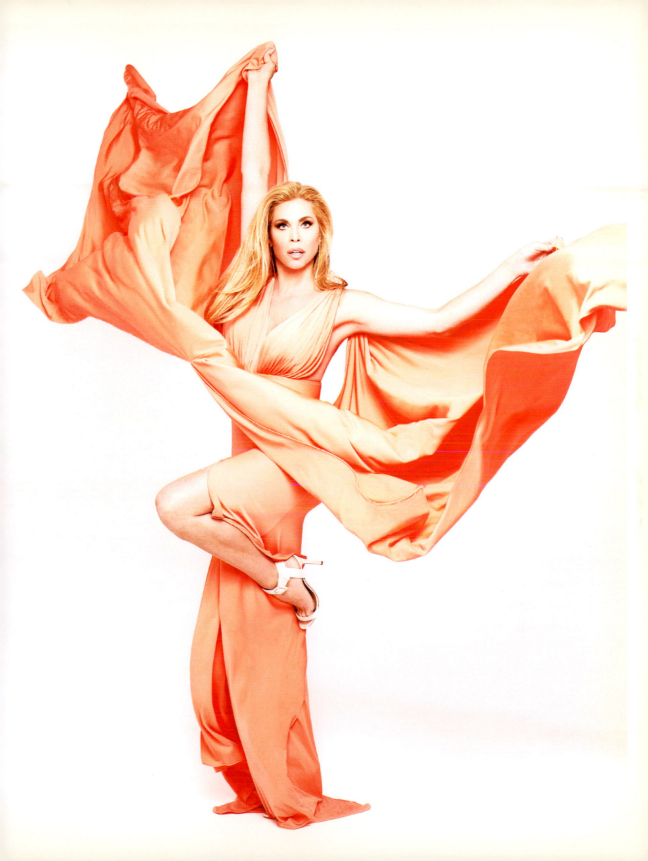

on to the next hurdle—tackling online dating. For a smokin' hot selfie-star like you, it shouldn't be too intimidating. Remember: online dating is the ultimate way to meet people when you're too busy to sit in coffee shops and wait for Prince or Princess Charming to show up and order you a pumpkin spice latte. So, what are the dos and don'ts, and how do you stay safe and keep your heart protected while surfing the 'net for your Mr. or Mrs. Right?

- Stay positive, upbeat, and patient. It takes time to meet the right one, especially if you're searching for love online.
- Make sure your profile is on point. Select a pro-pic that really captures your truest, brightest essence. For supplemental photos, pick the ones where you're at your happiest. Showcase your smiles in different activities. If your pro-pic is a mirror selfie, then make sure your supplemental pics are in different locations doing different things. Variety is key.
- Show a little more than you tell. The most successful profiles are the ones where your story is short, but your photos show a little more of your personality (and body). I'm not saying to go full-on Playboy shoot, but don't be afraid to show a little bit of shoulder or even some cleavage.
- Don't let your friends photobomb. Hey, you're putting yourself out there— not them.

- Don't confuse your future honey by putting too many crowded photos on your page.
- Be as honest as possible. Nobody likes to find out the person they chose to meet is nothing like they said they were in their profile. Honesty is most appreciated by those who themselves are honest, and isn't that what you want to attract?

Most important, keep it public. At least for the first few meetings, until you're sure this person isn't a creeper. If it turns out to be too close for comfort, go ahead and block the person, because your safety is 100 percent more important.

NAIL THAT INTERVIEW

There's another kind of "date" for you to get ready for, and it's called a job interview. It's a two-way street, because you should be checking out the company as much as they are checking you out. Here's my advice for interviews (and auditions, for that matter): Wear solid, power colors that complement your skin tone and hair color. Keep your shoes to a comfortable height (stilettoes are not ideal, but heels are great). Layer your look with a jacket so you can adjust to the temperature inside the office where you'll be interviewing. Instead of a superfeminine bag, consider dropping your wallet and lipstick into a high-quality leather messenger bag or briefcase. Limit your accessories to a few good pieces that are eye-catching without being distracting. And smile, because you are so worth the time and energy of all this preparation.

Walk confidently, and don't slouch. Slouching is a way of making yourself appear smaller (read: inferior), and that is not okay. You have every right to be there, sweetie, so put one foot in front of the other, and hold your head up high. Be proud of yourself for getting this far!

I have a friend who is in the career coaching business, and she always says the people who score highest in interviews are the ones who are best in the art of being themselves. That is absolutely true. The more "real" you are to your interviewer(s), the more likely you are going to get a callback for a second interview—or even an offer. People like people who are comfortable in their own skin, and it's inspiring to

them because so many of us are not. Discomfort equals a lack of confidence, at least in an interviewer's mind, so practice your breathing skills, and do your best to come across as real and confident and comfortable as you can command yourself to be.

A FINISHING TOUCH CHECK

So you've worked your way through all of the fabulous tips and tutorials in this book (which I've had so much fun sharing with you!), and now it's time for you to go out and present the real, more authentic you to the rest of the world. Sure, you are better looking than ever, from head to toe, but you're missing one more thing: a last-minute check in the mirror of your soul.

"Candis, I already looked in the mirror, and I look great!" you protest.

"Yes, sweetheart, you do, but what about the inside? Does it match the outside you?"

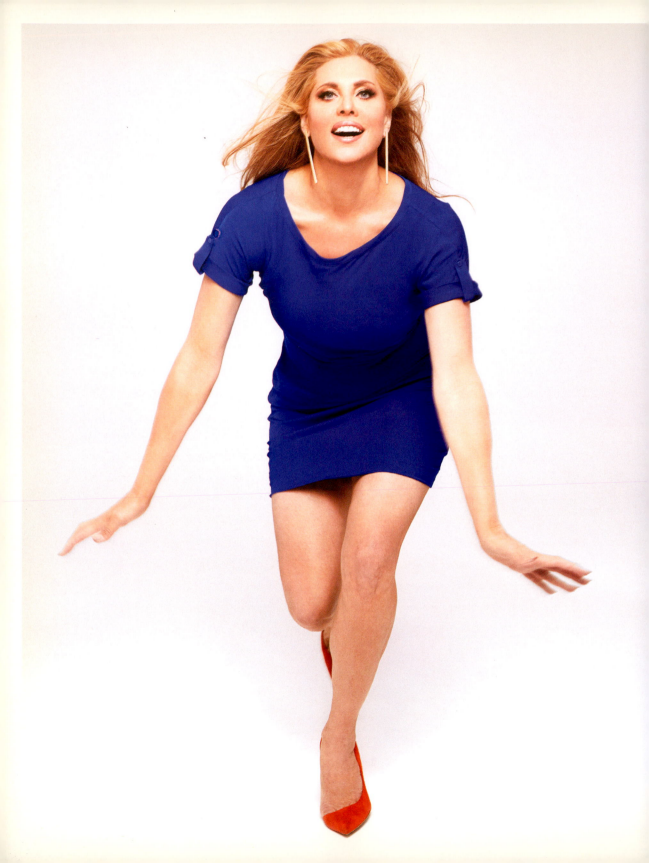

Before you close this book and head out the door, I'm going to ask you a few final questions:

❑ Have you stopped feeling "worth less" and started honoring yourself more?
❑ Have you accepted and embraced your flaws, and perhaps even learned how to use them to your advantage?
❑ Have you stopped body-shaming yourself and others? Have you helped others stop doing it as well?
❑ Have you found (and celebrated) your inner radiance?
❑ Have you broadened your own definition of what beauty is, who has it, and why?
❑ Have you felt yourself grow as a human being as a result of all your inner and outer work?

If you answered "yes" to all or most of these questions, you have so much to celebrate about yourself. You've come a long way—and though I may have helped, it was mostly through your own effort, just opening your eyes wide enough to see the beauty in everything.

This book happened because I understand how hard it can be to start over, to create confidence from nothing and to keep fighting for all that life can offer. More than many, I know the odds of finding your true radiance.

A few months ago, a little girl walked up to me and said, "Wow, Candis, you're so beautiful!" and I said to her, "You are so beautiful, too!" She really was gorgeous, but she said, "No, no, I'm not—not like you," and I thought, "Why doesn't she know this? What can I do to make her feel great about who she is?"

I wanted to write this book to inspire every woman of every gender, age, and race, to tell them that we are *all* beautiful. We just need to know it, allow it to become part of ourselves and our stories, with perhaps a little help to push us into realizing that with inner beauty comes outer beauty and that it is achievable for *everyone*.

Keep growing, and stay beautiful.

Xoxo,
Candis

CREATING A "VA-VA" VISION BOARD

Vision boards are a fantastic way for you to plan next year's look and attitude, like a professional stylist would!

Basically, this is creating a "mood board" for yourself—taking a holistic and very visual approach to goal-setting, so that you can get yourself on the fast track to the confident new you that's already (and always) in progress.

When I do my "Va-Va" Vision Board, I like to set aside at least half a day, and set the mood as positively as possible with some inspiring music (get up and dance in the middle of it, to celebrate!).

Starting with a large poster board that you can divide into four quadrants that represent each side of yourself that you present to others, let's meditate on a few important questions for each as we grab some scissors, glue, and a stack of your favorite fashion and lifestyle magazines and go to town.

Quadrant One: Personal

- Who are you now?
- What are your personal (psychological, relationship, spiritual) goals for this year?
- What word or words work best as your personal "theme" for the year?
- What is the color scheme you think best brings that theme to life?
- How are you planning to *shine* this year, with hair/makeup/fashion?

Quadrant Two: Career

- Where are you in your work life right now, and where would you like to be in the coming year?
- How can you dress for the job you want versus the one you have right now?
- What are your best "power" looks? Colors?
- What accessories will help you to feel stronger and more productive?

Quadrant Three: Social

- How do your friends currently see you? (Use words and images.)
- What fun goals do you and your friends have in the coming year? (Activities, trips, etc.)
- What looks (styles, colors, fabrics) best work with these goals?
- Are there outfits you can buy and trade or share with friends?

Quadrant Four: Global

- How do you see the world and your own unique place in it?
- What changes can you play a direct role in to make the world a better place?
- What one gift can you share with others?
- If you could travel anywhere in the world this year, where would it be and why? What would you wear, and how might traveling to this place influence your own style going forward?

In the center, you can put some keywords that best exemplify what your personal theme is for the year—or a quote or affirmation that accomplishes the same thing.

The whole idea is to create a vision board that builds on a theme and complements not only who you are now, but also who you'd like to be in the year ahead. When you're done, post it in your bedroom so that you can see it and reinforce your commitment to a better you. This is a great way to build your inner strength and confidence!

P. S. It's a good idea to hold onto each year's "Va-Va" Vision Board, since it will create a fashion timeline that tracks the evolution of your style. Fashion is cyclical, so you can easily see where you can take looks of the past into the future with just a few easy updates. Plus, it's fun to see how much you've changed over the years!

RESOURCES

Here are my favorites in each category!

Beauty Bloggers

Beauty is Boring (beautyisboring.com)

I Covet Thee (icovetthee.com)

Cult of Pretty (cultofpretty.com)

The Formula Blog (theformulablog.com)

A Model Recommends (amodelrecommends.com)

dizzybrunette3 (dizzybrunette3.com)

CurlyNikki (curlynikki.com)

Beauty Bets (beautybets.com)

Women's Style and Beauty Publications

InStyle

Vogue

Glamour

Cosmopolitan

Mademoiselle

Books

Workin' It! RuPaul's Guide to Life, Liberty, and the Pursuit of Style by RuPaul, It Books, 2010. An original, written by a true original. This book was written way before its time.

Your Beauty Mark: The Ultimate Guide to Eccentric Glamour by Dita Von Teese, Dey Street Books, 2015. Dita and collaborator Rose Apodaca take you through every step of Dita's glamour arsenal, and includes her confidantes—masters in makeup, hair, medicine, and exercise, as well as some of the world's most eccentric beauties—for authoritative advice.

Pretty Happy: Healthy Ways to Love Your Body by Kate Hudson, Dey Street Books, 2016. Hudson asserts that the key to living well, and healthy, is to plug into what your body needs, understanding that one size does not fit all, all the time, and being truly honest with yourself about your goals and desires. She focuses on exercise, making the right food choices, and not holding yourself to unrealistic standards of perfection.

Strong Looks Better Naked by Khloé Kardashian, Regan Arts, 2015. Kardashian writes with passion about the power of strength in spite of lifelong issues with body image. Filled with practical advice, recipes, and compelling personal anecdotes, *Strong Looks Better Naked* is a book informed by Khloé's own experiences. She emphasizes that a strong, properly cared for body is the foundation of a strong life.

Make Up: Your Life Guide to Beauty, Style, and Success—Online and Off by Michelle Phan, Harmony, 2014. From creating a gorgeous smoky eye to understanding contouring to developing an online persona, *Make Up* is packed with Michelle's trademark beauty and style tutorials, stories and pictures from her own life, plus advice on the topics she is asked about most, including etiquette, career, entrepreneurship, and creativity.

ABOUT THE MODELS

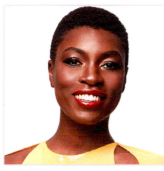

My name is **ASHIA TOKPONWEY** and I was born and raised in Brooklyn, New York, where I live with my longest friend, my dear cat Bubbles. As I get older, I love how I find new ways to define my beauty. I think true beauty is within yourself—loving the way you think and see yourself. If you love yourself at the core, then makeup and accessories are just an added bonus! It may not be an easy journey for everyone, but learning to love yourself in spite of your insecurities is absolutely gratifying. When I learned to love myself from the inside out, I felt similar to my favorite dessert: cake. When you put all the hard work in to the batter of a cake and get a sweet and fulfilling result, you can't wait to decorate it and show everyone! That's essentially me and makeup.

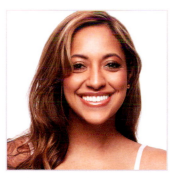

I am **CINDY DE LA HOZ**, a native of Philadelphia, PA and Colombian by heritage. I work as an editor and author of books on my favorite subjects: classic Hollywood, fashion, and empowering women's lifestyle like Candis's *Hi Gorgeous!* Among the books I've written are *So Audrey*, *A Touch of Grace*, and *Sophia Loren: Movie Star Italian Style*—all about women who have inspired me. I think of makeup as the artwork I do (almost) every day. I have fun with it! I also firmly believe that a little focus on self-care, beauty, and style can transform not just the way you look but how you feel, to present your most awesome self to the world.

ABOUT CANDIS'S DESIGNERS

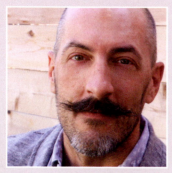

St. Louis native **CLAY G. SADLER** attended the International Academy of Merchandising and Design in Chicago. He developed his over-the-top and outrageous design aesthetic by designing evening gowns and costumes for some of the nation's most well-known female impersonators. Clay has made gowns and costumes for Candis Cayne for the past ten years, and is currently works with top fashion publications. As a graduate of the Fashion Institute of Design and Merchandising, Clay was invited to participate in the thirtieth anniversary celebration of the debut program and his works were shown at the Beverly Center in a week-long showing at center court. He has also worked with the fantastic the Best in Drag Show charity event for nearly a decade. The show raises funds for the Alliance for Housing and Healing (Aid for AIDs).

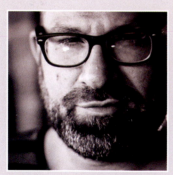

In 1994, **DAVID DALRYMPLE** began working with Patricia Field as the designer for the House of Field collection. David expanded and elevated the established lingerie-inspired fashion brand and celebrated the connection to New York's downtown scene. David's customer is not afraid to be the center of attention. Most notably, he designed the much-publicized nude illusion and Swarovski breakaway ensemble for Britney Spears that stopped the show at the 2000 MTV Video Music Awards. He has also dressed Pink, Mary J. Blige, Kim Cattrall, and Jennifer Lopez, just to name a few. He is committed to creating costumes, fashion, and his unique brand of sexy clothing in the historical garment center of New York City—producing only in the U.S., a challenge he finds extremely rewarding.

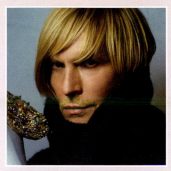

MARC BOUWER, who grew up in South Africa, had an unusual career trajectory. He was drafted into the army before studying fashion and winning the South African *Vogue* Young Designer award. His ambition drove him abroad. "There was only one place to go," he insists, "New York." His arrival, or what he calls his big "Hollywood moment," came when Halston studied his portfolio, then uttered six prophetic words: "I think you got something, kid." What Bouwer got was an offer to join Halston's studio. The Marc Bouwer aesthetic is the very definition of timeless elegance. The look is distinct—lush colors, plunging necklines, and daring up-to-there slits are undeniably sexy, yet kept in check by an appreciation for classic silver-screen glamour. In 2012, the Marc Bouwer Hybrid label was launched, a contemporary dress line represented by Joey Showroom, and available at retailers Saks Fifth Avenue and Anthropologie.

ACKNOWLEDGMENTS

This book is a dream that became a reality because of the following people: my manager, John Sobanski; agent Frank Weimann of Folio Literary Management; my coauthor, Katina Z. Jones; editor Cindy De La Hoz; book designer Frances Soo Ping Chow, and the rest of the team at Running Press. I would also like to thank my wonderful parents for their love and support.

—Candis

Special thanks to my wonderful husband and best friend, John; my daughters, Lilly Romestant (for editorial help) and Maddi Yaceczko (for beauty tips); and my agent, Frank Weimann, for his confidence and support over the past few decades.

—Katina